Speech and Language
Disorders in Multiple Sclerosis

Speech and Language Disorders in Multiple Sclerosis

EDITED BY
BRUCE E MURDOCH PhD
AND
DEBORAH G THEODOROS PhD

Department of Speech Pathology and Audiology,
The University of Queensland, Brisbane

W

WHURR PUBLISHERS

LONDON AND PHILADELPHIA

© 2000 Whurr Publishers
First published 2000 by
Whurr Publishers Ltd
19b Compton Terrace, London N1 2UN, England
325 Chestnut Street, Philadelphia PA 1906, USA

British Library Cataloguing in Publication Data
A catalogue record for this book is available from the British
Library.

ISBN 1 86156 100 8

Printed and bound in the UK by Athenaeum Press Ltd,
Gateshead, Tyne & Wear

Contents

Contributors

Lena Hartelius PhD   Götenborg University
                                    Sweden

Fiona J Hinchliffe PhD   The University of Queensland
                                    Australia

Jennifer B Lethlean PhD   Princess Alexandra Hospital, Brisbane
                                    Australia

Bruce E Murdoch PhD   The University of Queensland
                                    Australia

Deborah G Theodoros PhD   The University of Queensland
                                    Australia

Elizabeth C Ward PhD   The University of Queensland
                                    Australia

Preface

Ever since the first description of multiple sclerosis appeared in 1877, it has been recognized that a deficit in communicative abilities is an important part of the symptom complex of multiple sclerosis. Until recently, however, little attention has been given to further delineation of the neuropathophysiological basis and nature of these communicative impairments. In fact, it is only in the past decade that it has been recognized that multiple sclerosis can be associated with the occurrence of language disturbance in addition to the more widely recognized motor speech disorders. For most of the past century, the little research that has attempted to define further the features of the communicative impairments observed in persons with multiple sclerosis, has focused almost exclusively on the associated dysarthria.

However, even that research has been limited in its scope, being restricted primarily to studies based on perceptual analyses of dysarthria in multiple sclerosis, with little research being devoted to the further understanding of the physiological bases of the motor speech impairment exhibited by patients with this condition. Chapters 4–6 of the current book represent the first occasion on which the findings of a comprehensive physiological examination of the various subcomponents of the speech production apparatus in persons with multiple sclerosis have been published. The need for research of this type is highlighted by the current lack of effective and long-lasting intervention strategies for the treatment of motor speech impairments in multiple sclerosis. Chapter 6 of the current book addresses this issue in particular and provides directions for clinicians to take when treating speech disorders in multiple sclerosis, based on sound physiological analyses of the motor speech impairment.

As we enter the new millennium, there has never in the history of mankind been a greater emphasis placed on the need for good communication skills. As editors of the current book, we believe that it is therefore timely that attention be given to the communicative impairments exhibited by persons with multiple sclerosis. In many cases, the inability of persons with multiple sclerosis to communicate effectively with their families, their colleagues and the broader community, represents the most significant factor in their disability, leading in many instances to loss of vocational standing and social isolation. The need for further research into the nature of communicative impairments in multiple sclerosis, therefore, is urgent and the current book represents the first attempt to draw attention to the communication impairments exhibited by persons afflicted with multiple sclerosis. In particular, the addition of the chapters devoted to the documentation of the presence of language impairments in multiple sclerosis is seen by the editors as crucial to alerting speech pathologists, medical practitioners and other relevant health professionals to the long neglected problems in language function experienced by many persons with this condition. It is our hope that the contents of Chapters 7 through to 10 of the present text will provide speech pathologists with guidance to the nature of these language problems and alert them to the potential needs of their clients with multiple sclerosis in this area.

The editors wish to thank the numerous people with multiple sclerosis who, despite their disabilities, attended the necessary testing sessions which provided the data base for Chapters 2–9. We also wish to acknowledge the National Multiple Sclerosis Society of Australia for their generous financial support of our research.

Bruce E Murdoch
Deborah G Theodoros

Chapter 1
Neuropathophysiological basis of communication disorders in multiple sclerosis

BRUCE E MURDOCH

Introduction

Multiple sclerosis (MS) has been defined as 'an acquired primary demyelinating disease of the central nervous system (CNS) in which myelin is the target of an autoimmune inflammatory process(es)' (Whitaker and Mitchell, 1997, p. 4). Its clinical manifestations typically appear between 20 and 40 years of age with focal, multifocal, episodic and general neurological symptoms and signs. Although the presence of a speech disorder was included in the triad of symptoms described by Charcot as being pathognomic of MS in the first clinical description of the condition in 1877, until recently little attention has been paid by researchers to the communicative impairments exhibited by sufferers of MS. Further, it is now recognized that in addition to speech impairments, disturbances in cognitive-linguistic function are also manifest in some persons with MS. The aim of the current book is to provide a synthesis of current knowledge relating to communication disorders associated with MS and to outline procedures for the assessment and treatment of these disorders. The contents will cover not only the more widely recognized motor speech disorders seen in association with MS but also the more recently recognized cognitive-linguistic deficits exhibited by patients with this condition.

The present chapter reviews the neuropathophysiology, epidemiology, aetiology and clinical manifestations of MS and provides a basic introduction to the associated communication disorders. The medical treatments applied to MS are also described. Subsequent chapters of the current book are devoted to detailed analyses of the various speech and cognitive-linguistic impairments seen in MS together with a description of appropriate assessment and treatment strategies.

1

Neuropathophysiology of multiple sclerosis

MS is a disease of the white matter of the CNS, characterized by dissemi-nated demyelination of neuronal axons within the CNS with relative preservation of axon integrity (Raine, 1977). Myelin is an insulative lipid that encircles neuronal axons throughout the nervous system, in a sheath-like fashion (Sherwood, 1993). The myelin is manufactured by independent central and peripheral nervous system myelin-producing cells, oligodendrocytes in the CNS and Schwann cells in the peripheral nervous system, and provides a high resistance, low-capacitance insula-tion for the axon. In the unimpaired nervous system, the myelin produced is characteristically segmented into discrete units along each axon, separated by nodes of Ranvier (Hashimoto and Paty, 1986). Myelinated axons conduct nerve impulses from node to node in a salta-tory, rather than a continuous manner, which allows a reduction in conduction time and an increased metabolic efficiency. It is not surprising therefore that demyelination, as occurs in MS, is accompanied by significant conduction abnormalities (Kocsis and Waxman, 1985). Eisen (1983) stated that the pathophysiological hallmark of demyelina-tion is slow conduction, attributed to a reduction in ionic shift propaga-tions along bare axonal segments.

Demyelination of normally myelinated tracts within the CNS occurs in a periaxial fashion in MS with little or no axonal degeneration (van Oosten et al., 1995). Irregular grey islands known as 'plaques' are often seen at autopsy in regions where demyelination has occurred, particu-larly in the optic nerves, pons, medulla oblongata, spinal cord, cerebellum, the superior surface of the corpus callosum and the periven-tricular regions of the cerebral hemispheres (De Souza, 1990; Matthews et al., 1991). Although MS appears to have a predilection for certain sites within the CNS, no myelinated tract within the brain or spinal cord is exempt from attack (Hallpike et al., 1983). The anatomical distribution of lesions is highly variable between individuals, and within any one case plaques may vary considerably in size, shape and age (Matthews et al., 1991).

The demyelination process has been described as phasic, involving the progression of an acute lesion to a chronic plaque (Hashimoto and Paty, 1986). It has been hypothesized that the acute lesion is the result of an inflammatory reaction, involving the infiltration of inflammatory cells (primarily lymphocytes, plasma cells and macrophages) through the blood-brain barrier. These cells accumulate at the site of demyelination and engulf the degenerating myelin (van Oosten et al., 1995). As the lesion becomes chronic, reactive gliosis (formation of scar tissue as a result of astrocyte proliferation) occurs and inflammatory activity becomes less marked, resulting in the formation of the typical 'sclerotic plaque'. Accompanying the formation of these plaques, the myelin sheaths and oligodendrocytes are lost, and axonal loss also tends to occur, especially in severe, long-standing cases of MS (van Oosten et al., 1995).

It is now generally accepted that remyelination (i.e. the process in which demyelinated axons are re-invested with new myelin sheaths) does occur in the CNS and may contribute to lasting recovery from acute relapse in some cases of MS (Scolding and Franklin, 1998). However, in MS this remyelination process is far from complete and myelin repair ultimately fails during progression of the disease, as disability and handicap accumulate. As yet, however, the factors which limit the oligodendritic remyelination process are not understood (Allen, 1991).

Epidemiology and aetiology of multiple sclerosis

The aetiology of MS is unknown. Currently MS is classified as a T-cell-mediated organ-specific autoimmune disease (Martin and McFarland, 1995). Although evidence acquired from MS patients has supported the autoimmune theory, current thinking regarding the possible aetiology of MS has largely been shaped by studies based on experimental models of CNS inflammation, especially experimental allergic encephalomyelitis. Characteristically, the onset of symptoms of MS occurs post-pubescently, with peak incidence rates occurring between 30 and 40 years of age (De Souza, 1990). Onset of symptoms after 60 years of age is rare (Acheson, 1985). There is general agreement that MS is slightly more common in females than males, with female to male ratios reported to be in the order of 1.5:1 (Hartelius et al., 1995). Acheson (1985) attributed this female predilection to a possible hormonal interaction. Furthermore, the global distribution of MS illustrates characteristic latitudinal and racial profiles which have provided impetus for the development of numerous environmental and genetic theories of causation (Hashimoto and Paty, 1986).

It is generally accepted that MS is more common in countries further from the equator, both in the northern and southern hemispheres, with the peak prevalence rates having been documented in Caucasian populations residing at latitudes between 40° and 60° (Rivera, 1986). Specific regions of peak prevalence (i.e. greater than or equal to fifty cases per 100,000 population) include: northern and central Europe, northern North America, New Zealand and parts of Southern Australia (Hashimoto and Paty, 1986). MS prevalence rates in Australia comply with the latitudinal patterns of the northern hemisphere, with prevalence increasing with distance from the equator. MS has been reported to be four times more common in Tasmania (75.6 cases per 100,000) than in Queensland (18.6 cases per 100,000) (McLeod et al., 1994).

According to Compston (1994), the uneven geographical distribution associated with MS may indirectly reflect underlying environmental factors of causation. Postulated environmental influences have included nutrition, diet, agricultural production, sanitation, geological environment (e.g. presence/absence of trace elements) (Bauer and Hanefeld, 1993), infectious agents (e.g. viruses, spirochetes, mycoplasma) (Dick, 1976), as well as climate and social customs (Hutter, 1993). The strongest evidence to support an environmental pathogenesis has come from the results of migration studies which have shown that living at higher latitudes during childhood and adolescence increases a person's susceptibility to MS in adult life (Hutter, 1993). Further, documented trends indicate that migration prior to the age of 15 promotes the acquisition of the risk rate of the individual's new environment; however, birth place risk levels are maintained if migration occurs after 15 years of age (Kurtzke, 1983a). Based on these observations, many researchers investigating the possible cause of MS have hypothesized that an environmental agent (possibly a slow virus endemic to temperate climates) present prior to the age of 15 may be responsible for the subsequent manifestation of this disease (Tienari, 1994).

In a recent review, however, Poser (1994) questioned the viability of the often-cited interrelation between prevalence and latitude, in that prevalence of MS varies enormously in populations living on the same latitude. Poser (1994) concluded that genetic susceptibility plays a much more significant part than geography in determining the prevalence of MS in a particular location, although the degree and complexity of genetic control remains largely undefined (Sadovnick, 1994). Currently, there is growing support among MS researchers for the hypothesis that one or more environmental agents trigger the disease in a genetically susceptible host resulting in immune-mediated tissue injury within the CNS (Cook et al., 1995). Although the potency of various environmental factors in influencing the expression of MS is unknown, a non-specific infectious agent or agents, socio-economic factors and diet are thought to contribute (Hutter, 1993; Poser, 1994).

A number of viruses have been reported to cause demyelination in both humans (e.g. subacute sclerosing panencephalitis) and animals (e.g. canine distemper demyelinating encephalomyelitis) (Meulen and Stephenson, 1983). As such, viral-driven aetiological hypotheses have been applied to manifestations of MS (Meulen and Stephenson, 1983). Serological studies of blood serum and cerebrospinal fluid (CSF) in MS patients have revealed characteristically high antibody titres for measles, and less commonly, elevated titres for rubella, mumps, varicella, herpes, paramyxovirus and human T-cell leukaemia virus 1, among others (Bauer and Hanefeld, 1993). A distinctive CSF antibody triad of elevated measles, rubella and zoster antigens, was documented in up to 80% of an MS subject sample studied by Felgenhauer et al. (1985). Dick (1976) hypothesized that the MS-initiating viral agent, most probably acquired during childhood, lies dormant within the CNS until adolescence. Post-pubescently the virus is 'awakened' by unidentified stimuli, to precipitate a demyelinating rampage. Hashimoto and Paty (1986) suggested that this post-viral demyelination is immune mediated.

A viral aetiopathogenesis is supported by habitually elevated levels of specific immunoglobulins in the CSF of MS patients (Dick, 1976). Hashimoto and Paty (1986) stated that the immune system operates on the premise of an antigen-specific control response to foreign agents. Numerous abnormalities of immune regulation have been identified in MS patients including: virus-specific, antibody producing plasma cells surrounding areas of demyelination; production of high levels of CSF immunoglobulins, specifically IgG; and most strikingly, the loss of suppressor T-lymphocyte cells from the blood, prior to relapse (Rivera, 1986). This characteristic immunological profile may be indicative of a viral reaction, delayed hypersensitivity to viral antigens, or an autoimmune response (Leibowitz, 1983). The manifestation of MS in selective hosts subsequent to various viral infections may be attributed to a genetic susceptibility (Tienari, 1994). Ebers (1992) remarked that MS may be feasibly accepted as an autoimmune disease, under genetic influences.

Although MS occurs in all three of the principal racial groups of the world comprising Caucasoid (white), Mongoloid (oriental) and Negroid (black) populations, not all racial groups appear to be equally susceptible to the disease. In general it appears that MS is most common in caucasian populations but rare in oriental, negroid (Tienari, 1994), Australian Aboriginal and Torres Strait Islander populations (McLeod et al., 1994). Even when residing in high-risk locations, these latter ethnic groups manifest lower than expected prevalence rates for MS suggesting that they may be protected against the disease by some racially determined genetic factor (Hashimoto and Paty, 1986). Further evidence of a genetic influence in the occurrence of MS comes from studies that have shown that first degree relatives of affected individuals are 25–50 times more likely to develop MS than the general population (Wikstrom et al., 1984; Sadovnick et al., 1992). In addition, twin studies have documented concordance rates in monozygotic and dizygotic twins of 25% and 3% respectively, highly suggestive of a genetic influence (Ebers et al., 1986).

The human leukocyte antigen (HLA) gene complex on chromosome 6 is associated with immune functions (Tienari, 1994). Representations of certain loci on this gene complex have been characteristically linked to autoimmune diseases, including MS (Hauser et al., 1989). Of note, dissimilarities in HLA associations have been identified between different racial groups (Acheson, 1985), and as such, the isolation of a universal MS susceptibility gene cannot be substantiated. Despite these variable findings, however, histocompatibility antigen studies have given indisputable validity to the genetic theory of causation (Batchelor, 1985).

In essence, it appears that we cannot sequester the aetiological agents responsible for the manifestation of MS. The combined effects of genetic and environmental influences provide us with the most viable interpretation of the neuropathology associated with MS (Poser, 1994). It has been postulated that a genetic susceptibility predisposes the individual to disease acquisition; however, environmental elements of unknown origin are thought to be responsible for activating the onset of clinical symptoms (Poser, 1994).

Clinical manifestations of multiple sclerosis

The clinical signs and symptoms associated with MS vary tremendously from case to case as a consequence of the variability in the anatomic distribution and age of the CNS lesions. Despite the fact that demyelination may occur virtually anywhere within the CNS, the majority of patients with MS have their initial symptoms in a relatively limited distribution. McAlpine (1972) documented limb weakness, optic neuritis, paraesthesia in the extremities, diplopia, vertigo and impaired micturition to be the most common primary clinical manifestations of MS. Dysarthria, dysphagia, nystagmus, auditory dysfunction, weakness, ataxia, intention tremor, spasticity, sphincter disturbances and altered emotional responses are symptoms that manifest more commonly in patients with long-standing or advanced MS. Pain is not usually a presenting symptom of MS but frequently develops during the course of the illness in such forms as trigeminal neuralgia and pseudoradicular pain. Generalized fatigue subsequent to increases in body temperature or episodes of physical exertion is also frequently seen in MS, and may be of a persistent or transient nature (Bauer and Hanefeld, 1993). Fatigue has been noted to result in reduced motivation levels and decreased work performance.

Transient symptoms known as paroxysmal attacks are commonly experienced in MS, especially in the early stages of the disease (Mitchell, 1993). These attacks are usually brief and intense, lasting seconds to minutes, and with a tendency to recur in a stereotypic manner for each individual (Matthews et al., 1991). Paroxysmal dysarthria and ataxia have both been frequently reported as the most common type of paroxysmal attacks. Other paroxysmal disorders associated with MS include trigeminal neuralgia, tonic seizures and spasms, and unpleasant quivering sensations (Mitchell, 1993).

The general course of MS is variable and may take several forms including: relapsing-remitting; progressive-relapsing; and chronically progressive. Approximately 65% of individuals with MS experience a relapsing-remitting form of the disease at onset, with symptoms usually developing subacutely and resolving over weeks to months, with the periods between disease relapses being characterized by a lack of disease progression (Mitchell, 1993). After a varying number of exacerbations a majority of the individuals with relapsing-remitting MS also enter a secondary progressive phase where symptoms gradually evolve without remission. Progressive-relapsing MS occurs in about 15% of patients and represents a progressive disease from outset, with clear acute relapses, with or without full recovery, with periods between relapses characterized by continuing progression. The chronically progressive form of MS exists in approximately 20% of patients and is characterized by disease progression from outset with only occasional plateaus and temporary minor improvements.

Diagnosis of MS is difficult and typically made by exclusion, with heavy reliance on clinical history and neurological symptoms using the criteria specified by Poser et al. (1983). These criteria are based on dissemination in time and space and the diagnostic categories include *definite*, *probable* and *possible* MS. For a definite diagnosis, clinical evidence of lesions in two or more functional systems is needed (Poser et al., 1983). Confirmatory evidence can also be gained by the use of Magnetic Resonance Imaging (MRI), cerebrospinal fluid analysis and multisensory evoked potentials (Rao, 1986). Probable MS is specified in cases where relapsing-remitting symptoms are present with only one neurological sign commonly associated with MS. A diagnosis of *possible* MS is made where relapsing-remitting symptoms are present without documented signs or objective signs are insufficient to establish more than one site of CNS involvement. Although the diagnosis of MS is far easier and more certain with the availability of cranial MRI, a determination of disease activity and the disease progression remains difficult.

Medical treatment of multiple sclerosis

Effective curative therapy for MS is as yet unavailable. Consequently, medical management of MS continues to focus on the treatment of acute exacerbations, prevention of relapse and progression, and alleviation of the chronic symptoms of the disease (Noseworthy, 1991; Francis, 1993; van Oosten et al., 1995). Acute exacerbations are principally treated with drugs such as corticosteroids that possess properties that accelerate the recovery that usually follows each attack (Rudick and Goodkin, 1992;

Ebers, 1994). Most neurologists limit the use of these drugs to only the most serious or disabling episodes (Francis, 1993) since long-term administration does not alter the natural history of the disease significantly and moreover, steroid side-effects outweigh this limited benefit (Ebers, 1994). The corticosteroids, corticotrophin (adrenocorticotrophic hormone, ACTH) and methylprednisolone have been reported to accelerate recovery from relapse in MS equally well (Thompson et al., 1989), although their effects are probably only short-lived (Barkhof et al., 1994). Methylprednisolone is usually the preferred treatment option because it has the convenience of a shorter treatment course (Mitchell, 1993; van Oosten et al., 1995). Another treatment sometimes used in cases of acute exacerbation, especially in pregnant patients (Mitchell, 1993), is plasma exchange. This treatment produces only minimal benefits which fail to justify the cost (Weiner et al., 1989).

As a result of current thoughts on MS pathogenesis, the drugs used to prevent relapse and slow progression of the disease are typically immunosuppressive agents (Francis, 1993). Immunosuppressive drugs such as azathioprine, cyclophosphamide and cyclosporin may slow the progression of MS to some degree; however, potentially serious adverse side-effects including hypertension, anaemia and gastrointestinal complications have limited their use.

Interferon beta (IFN-B) has recently been demonstrated to be of value in reducing relapses and preventing the accumulation of brain lesions over time in MS, without producing serious adverse side-effects (Jacobs et al., 1994; Jacobs and Johnson, 1994). Generally, the interferons act to stimulate the immune system, activating macrophages, enhancing natural killer cells and inhibiting virus replication (Francis, 1993). Interferon beta has not yet been observed to have an effect on the accumulation of disability over time (Jacobs et al., 1994). Another recently investigated treatment involving co-polymer 1 (COP 1) administered daily to patients via subcutaneous injections has shown modest benefits in slowing the progression of both the relapsing-remitting and progressive forms of MS (Francis, 1993; Jacobs et al., 1994).

The symptomatic treatment of MS involves a wide variety of pharmacological agents. Spasticity is experienced frequently in established MS and is most commonly treated with anti-spastic agents such as baclofen, tizandine, diazepam and dantrolene carefully titrated to provide relief of spasticity without either producing or exacerbating muscular weakness (van Oosten et al., 1995). Unfortunately, specific treatment is unavailable to combat the disabling effects of muscle weakness (van Oosten et al., 1995).

Ataxia is also a relatively frequent and disabling symptom of MS which is difficult to treat (van Oosten et al., 1995). Most agents used for the problem of ataxia have only a damping effect on incapacitating tremor, with the likelihood of tolerance to the drug(s) developing, as well as the production of unacceptable side-effects (Francis, 1993). Fatigue has the potential to impact profoundly on daily living in patients with MS. Amantadine and pemoline are often used to lessen the physiological component of fatigue but the psychological component requires counselling and sometimes the administration of antidepressant drugs (Francis, 1993). Urinary tract symptoms such as detrusor hyperreflexia and abnormally high postmicturitional volumes, are generally treated using oral anticholinergic medication and intermittent self-catheterization (van Oosten et al., 1995).

Much controversy surrounds the efficacy of currently used MS therapies due to difficulties in determining whether stabilization of a patient's condition has occurred spontaneously or as a response to therapy. Although many therapies have been reported to be effective based on limited trials or following initial application, many have been found later to provide no benefit on the basis of larger trials or after the passage of time (Mitchell, 1993).

Individuals with MS have complex problems and the potential for significant and sometimes severe disability despite the currently used treatments. In view of this, many authors (Noseworthy, 1991; Mitchell, 1993) advocate a multidisciplinary approach to the treatment of MS to provide patients with optimal care. Physical, occupational, speech and recreational therapy are all important in assisting MS patients to experience a good quality of life. Communicative impairment, resulting from the presence of a significant dysarthria, may be an important contributor to a reduction in the quality of life for some individuals with MS. Ultimately, both medical and rehabilitative therapies should be tailored to suit each patient's individual needs (Mitchell, 1993).

Introduction to speech and language disorders in multiple sclerosis

Although the presence of a speech disorder is a commonly reported symptom of MS, traditionally the disease has been considered to have little impact on cognitive-linguistic abilities. The findings of recent studies, however, suggest that the prevalence of cognitive-linguistic impairments in MS have been underestimated, the low prevalence reported in earlier studies having been attributed to the use of inappropriate and insufficiently sensitive tests of language ability.

Dysarthria in multiple sclerosis

Dysarthria is the most common communication disorder affecting individuals with MS (Beukelman et al., 1985). Dysarthria has been defined as 'a collective name for a group of speech disorders resulting from disturbances in muscular control over the speech mechanism due to damage of the central or peripheral nervous system. It designates problems in oral communication due to paralysis, weakness or incoordination of the speech musculature' (Darley et al., 1969a, b p. 246). The definition implies that dysarthria may affect the speed, strength, range, timing or accuracy of speech movements involved in the speech processes of respiration, phonation, nasality, articulation and prosody (speech rate, stress, and intonation), singly or in combination. Although recognized as a frequently occurring symptom of MS, the dysarthria exhibited by persons with this disease has received little attention from researchers in this field. While neurology textbooks invariably make reference to the presence of dysarthria in MS, in general they fail to provide detailed descriptions of the disorder, and consequently the nature of the speech disturbance has remained relatively poorly understood.

The French neurologist Charcot (1877) provided the first description of the perceptual features of MS dysarthria. He considered dysarthria to be one of three cardinal symptoms of MS (together with nystagmus and intention tremor) and described the motor speech disorder as follows:

> The affected person speaks in a slow, drawling manner, and sometimes almost unintelligibly. It seems as if the tongue had become 'too thick', and the delivery recalls that of an individual suffering from incipient intoxication. A closer examination shows that the words are as if measured or scanned; there is a pause after every syllable, and the syllables are pronounced slowly (pp.192–3).

Since Charcot's original description, three different methods have been used by researchers in the characterization of different aspects of dysarthria, including dysarthria in MS. These methods include perceptual methods (careful auditory evaluation of speech characteristics, often using specifically chosen parameters and rating scales), physiological methods (involving the use of a range of specialized physiological instruments to assess the functioning of the major components of the speech production mechanism) and acoustic methods (studying aspects of the acoustic speech signal as reflections of the speaker's disordered speech movement patterns). The findings of the various studies based on perceptual, acoustic and physiological analyses of MS dysarthria are described and discussed in detail in Chapters 2–5 of this book. Chapter 6 provides a comprehensive overview of the treatments that can be applied to the motor speech disorders manifest in persons with MS.

Language disorders in multiple sclerosis

Until recently, research into communication problems in MS tended to concentrate on the motor aspects of speech rather than the possible language problems resulting from subcortical white matter demyelination. Traditionally, cognitive-linguistic abilities were thought to be a function of the cerebral cortex and consequently it was assumed that disruption to these abilities in diseases of the white matter was unlikely. However, it is becoming increasingly evident that the part played by white matter pathways and subcortical structures in both cognitive and language functions may have been underestimated. Researchers now propose that disruption of subcortical and brainstem influence on the cerebral cortex in MS can be responsible for cortical dysfunction leading to cognitive and linguistic disorders in this population (Crosson, 1985; Alexander et al., 1987; Wallesch and Papagno, 1988; Lethlean and Murdoch, 1994a). In particular, neural white matter pathways connecting subcortical structures such as the basal ganglia and thalamus to the cortical language areas have been considered important in language function (Alexander et al., 1987). Cognitive impairments subsequent to MS are now known to span the entire spectrum and include deficits in memory, intelligence, information processing, abstract and conceptual reasoning and attention (Beatty and Monson, 1989; Blackwood et al., 1991; Rao et al., 1993; Ruchkin et al., 1994). Likewise in studies where appropriate and sufficiently sensitive language tests have been used, individuals with MS have been shown to exhibit language deficits in the areas of naming, comprehension of logic or grammatical constructions, word fluency, verbal reasoning, word definitions and the interpretation of absurdities, ambiguities and metaphors (Lethlean and Murdoch, 1993, 1994a). Chapters 7–9 of this book provide a detailed description and discussion of the language disorders noted to occur in individuals with MS in the context of the role of subcortical white matter pathways in language processing. Chapter 10 presents a review of contemporary treatments applicable to persons with MS presenting with language disorders.

PART 1
MOTOR SPEECH DISORDERS IN MULTIPLE SCLEROSIS

Chapter 2
Perceptual features of dysarthria in multiple sclerosis

DEBORAH G THEODOROS, BRUCE E MURDOCH AND
ELIZABETH C WARD

Introduction

The earliest description of abnormal speech observed in persons with MS
was made by Charcot in 1877 who described a dysarthric speech disturbance characterized by slow, drawling, 'scanning speech'. Indeed,
dysarthria has been identified clinically as the most common type of
communication disorder observed in the MS population (Beukelman et al.,
1985). In general, the speech disturbance associated with MS presents as a
mixed dysarthria, the characteristics of which are determined by the sites of
central nervous system involvement. The speech disturbance in MS has
been attributed solely to brainstem lesions (Kurtzke, 1970; Poser, 1978),
while others regard dysarthria in MS as an indication of cerebellar dysfunction (Grinker and Sahs, 1966; Hallpike et al., 1983). Darley et al. (1972), in
relating the speech characteristics of subjects with MS to different neurological groups, found that the dysarthria could not be solely attributed to
involvement of the cerebellum, as the dysarthric speech disturbance was
noted to alter and increase in level of severity with additional dysfunction
in other components of the central nervous system. Those MS subjects with
cerebral, cerebellar, and brainstem involvement were found to exhibit the
most severe dysarthric speech disturbances. Furthermore, Hartelius et al.
(1995) have suggested that the MS subjects with predominantly cerebral or
cerebellar involvement demonstrate the most abnormal speech symptoms
compared to those persons with brainstem or spinal involvement. Based
on perceptual and neurological evidence to date, it is generally accepted
that persons with MS are more likely to demonstrate either ataxic or spastic
dysarthria in isolation, or a mixed ataxic-spastic dysarthric speech disturbance (Duffy, 1995; Hartelius et al., 1999, 2000).

Dysarthria associated with MS has been found to occur at varying stages of the disease. Generally, this speech disturbance is uncommon in the initial stages (Matthews, 1991), and tends to occur as a later manifestation following involvement of additional motor systems (Darley et al., 1972). Paroxysmal attacks of dysarthria have been reported as initial symptoms of MS, and throughout the course of the disease (Espir et al., 1966; Matthews, 1975; Osterman and Westerberg, 1975; Netsell and Kent, 1976; Perks and Lascelles, 1976; Twomey and Espir, 1980). These attacks, which may occur a few times per day or up to several times an hour, are characterized by brief bouts of slurred speech which last for a few seconds, remit, and then reappear for an additional few seconds (Netsell and Kent, 1976; Twomey and Espir, 1980).

Incidence and severity of dysarthria in multiple sclerosis

Although Charcot (1877) originally included a speech disturbance in his triad of symptoms characterizing MS (nystagmus, scanning speech, and intention tremor), dysarthria is not a universal feature of MS symptomatology. Indeed, dysarthria has generally been identified in approximately 40% to 50% of individuals with MS with an incidence as low as 23% being reported in the literature (Darley et al., 1972; Beukelman et al., 1985; Hartelius et al., 1993; Hartelius and Svensson, 1994). The variations in the incidence of dysarthria in MS populations, however, appear to reflect the diverse nature of the populations selected for study (severity, duration, and stage of disease progression), the research designs implemented (perceptual rating scales, surveys, clinical diagnosis), and the differences in terminology used to define a dysarthric speech disturbance.

Darley et al. (1972), in the largest study of individuals with MS, identified dysarthria in 41% of 168 cases based on the overall impact of the subject's speech on the listener. The incidence of dysarthria in Swedish MS populations has been reported to be 45% and 47% in two cohorts of subjects, involving 77 and 30 individuals, respectively (Hartelius et al., 1993, 1999, 2000). The presence of dysarthria in these studies was determined according to each subject's overall speech abnormality. A similar incidence of dysarthria in persons with MS has been identified in an Australian study by FitzGerald et al. (1987), where 48% of the 23 subjects were found to be dysarthric based on their overall speech intelligibility level, with 83% of the total group demonstrating consonant imprecision. Recently, the authors of the present chapter have examined the perceptual characteristics of a further cohort of 33 subjects with MS according to the methodology used by FitzGerald et al. (1987). Of these 33 subjects with MS, 30% were considered to be dysarthric based on either their overall level of intelligibility and/or their precision of consonant articulation. When combined with the data from the study by FitzGerald et al. (1987), 52% of the 56 cases were found to exhibit speech disturbances based on the presence of defective articulation, with 29% of the total cohort demonstrating reductions in overall speech intelligibility. The frequency of occurrence and level of severity of deviant speech dimensions perceived to be present in the Australian cohort of subjects with MS are shown in Table 2.1.

Two major surveys of the incidence of speech and voice problems in MS populations have revealed inconsistent findings, despite the involvement of large subject numbers. In a Swedish survey conducted by Hartelius and Svensson (1994), 44% of 203 respondents with MS reported that they had experienced impairments in speech and voice since the onset of the disease. Furthermore, 16% of these cases indicated that their speech disorder constituted their greatest handicap. In contrast, an even larger survey of 656 persons with MS conducted in the United States of America revealed that only 23% of the respondents reported the presence of speech or other communication problems (Beukelman et al., 1985).

Despite some inconsistencies in the incidence of dysarthria in MS populations, the majority of evidence suggests that the severity of the dysarthric speech disturbance associated with MS is predominantly mild, with the speech disturbance increasing with greater and more widespread neurological involvement (Darley et al., 1972). In their study, Darley et al. (1972) found that 36% of their 69 dysarthric speakers demonstrated minimal to mild speech impairments with only 5% of the subjects exhibiting a moderate to severe dysarthria. Similar patterns of severity of dysarthria have been identified in both Swedish (Hartelius et al., 1993, 1999, 2000) and Australian populations (FitzGerald et al., 1987). Of the MS subjects with dysarthria, reported by Hartelius et al. (1999, 2000), 37% exhibited a mild to moderate dysarthria with a further 8% of the subjects demonstrating a moderate to severe dysarthric speech disturbance. In the combined cohort of Australian persons with MS, more than half of the subjects with reductions in overall intelligibility (56%) were considered to demonstrate only a mild decrease in intelligibility while 19% of these cases were perceived to exhibit a severe reduction in intelligibility. Clinicians, therefore, are likely to encounter a wide range of severity of dysarthria within the MS population, and in individual patients over time, with the level of severity dependent upon the degree of neurological involvement. Despite the relatively high prevalence of dysarthria in MS populations, limited research has been conducted to define and document the perceptual characteristics of the motor speech disturbance in this neurologically impaired population.

Table 2.1 Frequency of occurrence of deviant speech dimensions of Australian subjects with MS (N = 56)

Deviant speech dimension	Frequency of deviation in total sample (N=56)		Severity of deviation					
			Mild		Moderate		Severe	
	N	%	N	%	N	%	N	%
Variation of pitch	30	54	17	57	10	33	3	10
Pitch level	29	52	20	69	8	28	1	3
Breath support	29	52	19	66	6	21	4	13
Imprecise consonants	29	52	20	69	6	21	3	10
Harshness	25	45	19	76	3	12	3	12
General rate	24	43	13	54	7	29	4	17
General stress	23	41	12	53	7	30	4	17
Hypernasality	23	41						
Pitch steadiness	22	39	15	68	5	23	2	9
Phrase length	22	39	9	41	11	50	2	9
Hoarseness	22	39	17	77	5	23	0	0
Prolonged intervals	22	39	9	41	9	41	4	18
Variation of loudness	21	38	14	67	7	33	0	0
Intermittent breathiness	21	38	15	71	6	29	0	0
Audible inspiration	21	38	14	67	4	19	3	14
Maintenance of loudness	20	36	15	75	5	25	0	0
Maintenance of rate	20	36	18	90	2	10	0	0
Glottal fry	20	36	18	90	1	5	1	5
Strained-strangled	17	30	11	64	3	18	3	18
Forced inspiration/ expiration	17	30	10	59	4	23	3	18
Overall intelligibility	16	29	9	56	4	25	3	19
Loudness level	15	27	15	100	0	0	0	0
Prolonged phonemes	15	27	7	47	6	40	2	13
Imprecise vowels	14	25	12	86	0	0	2	14
Rate fluctuations	14	25	13	93	1	7	0	0
Pitch breaks	13	23	8	62	2	15	3	23
Excessive loudness variation	12	21	8	66	2	17	2	17
Wetness	9	16	8	89	0	0	1	11
Short rushes	8	14	8	100	0	0	0	0
Hyponasality	8	14						
Mixed nasality	5	9	4	80	1	20	0	0
Grunt	2	4	2	100	0	0	0	0

Perceptual assessment of speech production in multiple sclerosis

Studies which have investigated the perceptual characteristics of speech production in persons with MS have employed a variety of techniques developed to assess dysarthric speech output. These techniques have provided a description of specific deviant speech dimensions, an assessment of motor speech subsystem dysfunction, an evaluation of overall speech intelligibility, and clinical measures of maximum performance on respiratory, phonatory, and articulatory tasks.

Descriptive equal-interval rating scales as used by Darley et al. (1972) and FitzGerald et al. (1987) have been used to rate a subject's speech sample according to a number of speech dimensions associated with the various processes of speech production: respiration, phonation, resonance, articulation, and prosody. Speech dimensions rated according to the severity of dysfunction (e.g. breath support for speech) are assessed on a four-point scale, while those dimensions rated according to the frequency of their occurrence in the total speech sample (e.g. rate fluctuations) are evaluated on a five-point scale. A seven-point scale, with the middle point of four representing normal, is used to rate certain speech dimensions which may be rated on the same scale as being too high or too low (e.g. pitch level). A more simplified version of a perceptual rating scale, although a less discriminatory measure, is the forced choice nominal scale, which involves the rater selecting a descriptor that most closely describes the speech characteristic, from a limited number of options (Hartelius et al., 1993).

Quantifiable tests of intelligibility have also been used to assess the speech of persons with MS. The Assessment of Intelligibility of Dysarthric Speech (ASSIDS) (Yorkston and Beukelman, 1981), as used in the study conducted by the current authors, determines single word and sentence intelligibility, speaking rate, and the communication efficiency of adult dysarthric speakers. These measures provide quantifiable data which can be used to monitor the progression of speech impairment, as well as treatment efficacy. Assessment of motor speech subsystem dysfunction in persons with MS can been achieved using the Frenchay Dysarthria Assessment (FDA) (Enderby, 1983). This test provides a standardized evaluation of speech neuromuscular activity involving respiration, phonation, resonance, articulation, and speech-related reflex activity. Hartelius et al. (1993) reported on the development and utilization of a clinical dysarthria test for individuals with MS which consisted of 54 test items divided into six subtests relating to respiration, phonation, oral motor performance, articulation, prosody, and intelligibility. The test was found to be sufficiently sensitive to discriminate between non-dysarthric and dysarthric MS speakers and controls and to identify subclinical signs of subsystem dysfunction in the MS population. Clinical measures of maximum performance on a variety of respiratory, articulatory, and phonatory tasks have also been found to provide useful information concerning the speech production of persons with MS.

Perceptual speech characteristics associated with multiple sclerosis

Those studies which have utilized some or all of these perceptual assessments to investigate the perceptual speech characteristics of persons with MS have consistently identified deficits in the various processes of speech production (Farmakides and Boone, 1960; Darley et al., 1972; FitzGerald et al., 1987; Hartelius et al., 1993, 1999, 2000) (see Table 2.2). As previously mentioned, approximately 40–50% of the subjects investigated in the majority of these studies demonstrated dysarthric speech disturbances.

Deficits in respiration have been noted in both breath support and control for speech, while hypernasality would appear to be the predominant disorder of resonance noted in this group. Descriptions of phonatory disorders in the MS population have encompassed a wide spectrum of abnormal vocal features including harshness, breathiness, glottal fry, hoarseness, and a strained-strangled vocal quality. The diversity of deviant phonatory features would appear to reflect the widespread neurological involvement possible in this population, in that the abnormal vocal features are consistent with different forms of laryngeal function (hyper- and hypofunction), associated with varying sites of neurological damage. These findings support the conclusion made earlier by Darley et al. (1972) that the dysarthric speech disturbance in MS was not necessarily a result of only brainstem or cerebellar dysfunction as previously suggested (Grinker and Sahs, 1966; Kurtzke, 1970; Poser, 1978; Hallpike et al., 1983). In all perceptual studies of persons with MS, articulation has been noted to be impaired in a proportion of the subjects, with respect to the precision of consonants and vowels, phoneme length, and sudden, irregular articulatory breakdowns. A range of prosodic disturbances relating to rate of speech, stress and intonation, pitch and loudness level and control, and fluency of speech output have been readily identified in the MS population across these studies.

A comparison of the ten most frequently occurring deviant speech dimensions in the three major MS populations (Australia, Sweden and the United States of America) studied to date, has identified five abnormal speech features common to all three MS populations:

Table 2.2 Summary of perceptual speech characteristics in persons with MS as reported in the literature

Study	Respiration	Phonation	Resonance	Articulation	Prosody
Farmakides and Boone (1960) N = 82	• ↓ Control of exhalation	• Weak voice • ↓ Loudness	• Hypernasality	• Slurred and indistinct	• ↓ Pitch variation • ↓ Rate
Darley et al. (1972) N = 168	• ↓ Ventilation and support • ↑ Breathing rate	• Harshness • Breathiness	• Hypernasality	• Defective articulation • Sudden articulatory breakdowns	• Impaired loudness control • Impaired stress • ↓ Pitch control • Inappropriate pitch level
Hartelius et al. (1993) N = 30 Hartelius et al. (2000) N = 77	• ↓ Breath control and support	• Creakiness • Breathiness • Harshness	• Hypernasality	• Imprecise consonants • Irregular articulatory breakdowns	• ↓ Pitch and loudness variation • ↓ Rate • Short phrases • Inappropriate/ prolonged pauses • Impaired stress pattern • Inappropriate pitch level
Combined Australian Study (FitzGerald et al., 1987; MSRU study) N = 56	• ↓ Breath support	• Harshness • Hoarseness • Intermittent breathiness • Glottal fry • Strained-strangled quality	• Hypernasality	• Imprecise consonants and vowels • Prolonged phonemes	• ↓ Pitch variation • Inappropriate pitch level • ↓ Rate • Impaired stress • ↓ Pitch steadiness • Phrase length • Prolonged intervals • ↓ Loudness variation • Maintenance loudness and rate

* MSRU = Motor Speech Research Unit, The University of Queensland; ↓ = Decreased; ↑ = Increased

harshness; imprecise articulation/consonant production; impaired emphasis/stress patterns; impaired respiratory support; and impaired pitch variation/ control (see Table 2.3). Although hypernasality was found to be one of the ten most frequently occurring deviant features in the speech output of persons with MS in the American and Australian populations, this abnormal characteristic was not found to be as prevalent in the Swedish population. Of the five deviant speech characteristics common to all three populations, imprecise articulation/consonant production was the most frequently perceived dimension across the three groups, followed by harshness, impaired emphasis/stress patterns, impaired respiratory support for speech, and impaired pitch variation/control, in descending order of frequency.

The presence of a harsh vocal quality in persons with MS is indicative of hyperfunctional laryngeal behaviour. Such laryngeal function is consistent with spastic dysarthria, a common component of the mixed dysarthria associated with MS. Similarly, the impaired emphasis or abnormal stress patterns and impaired pitch variation evident in the speech output of persons with MS could reflect the ataxic component of the mixed dysarthria observed clinically in these individuals. Interestingly, the 'scanning speech' described by Charcot (1877), consistent with severe excess and equal syllable stress (FitzGerald et al., 1987), has not been found to be a consistent feature in the speech of individuals with MS. Indeed, Darley et al. (1972) identified 'scanning' speech in only 14% of their 168 subjects with MS. Similarly, this abnormal speech feature was perceived to be present in only 17% of the subjects in the combined Australian study.

The impaired respiratory support for speech commonly noted in subjects with MS may reflect a combination of reduced lung volumes, abnormal speech breathing patterns, and/or respiratory muscle weakness due to varying levels of neurological impairment. Although individuals with MS are more likely to exhibit the five abnormal speech features described above, various deviant perceptual speech features may be manifested in any one person at different time intervals, depending on the specific pathology and progress of the disease. Perceptual evaluation of speech production in persons with MS, therefore, must be conducted on an individual basis.

Speech intelligibility in multiple sclerosis

In general, specific measures of speech intelligibility in persons with MS have revealed mild reductions in word and sentence intelligibility for this neurologically disordered group. Hartelius et al. (1993) found that their MS group of 30 subjects achieved 96% intelligibility in both words and sentences compared to the control group's 100% and 98% intelligibility

Table 2.3 Ten most frequently occurring deviant speech dimensions in MS subjects across three different populations.

Darley et al. (1972) (N = 168)	Combined Australian Cohort (Fitzgerald et al., 1987 and MSRU study) (N = 56)	Hartelius et al. (2000) (N = 77)
Impaired loudness control (77%)	Impaired pitch variation (54%) *	Imprecision of consonants (92%) *
Harshness (72%) *	Inappropriate pitch level (52%)	Glottal fry (88%)
Defective articulation (46%) *	Impaired breath support (52%) *	Prolonged intervals (87%)
Impaired emphasis (39%) *	Imprecision of consonants (52%) *	Harshness (86%) *
Impaired pitch control (37%) *	Harshness (45%) *	Impaired stress pattern (83%) *
Reduced respiratory support (Decreased vital capacity) (35%) *	Impaired rate (43%)	Inappropriate loudness level (81%)
Hypernasality (24%)	Impaired stress pattern (41%) *	Impaired overall intelligibility (78%)
Inappropriate pitch level (24%)	Hypernasality (41%)	Impaired respiratory support (77%) *
Breathiness (22%)	Reduced pitch steadiness (39%)	Impaired rate (74%)
Sudden articulatory breakdowns (9%)	Reduced phrase length (39%)	Impaired pitch variation (69%) *

* = Common to all three studies

for words and sentences, respectively. The small differences evident in intelligibility levels between the groups probably reflect the fact that both dysarthric and non-dysarthric speakers had been included in the MS group, and that the majority of the dysarthric speakers were not severely impaired. When the percentage scores for intelligibility for the MS group were combined with ratings of intelligibility in reading and spontaneous speech, a measure of speaking rate, and various overall assessments of communicative disability, Hartelius et al. (1993) reported that the MS group and the dysarthric subgroup were both found to be significantly impaired in overall intelligibility compared to the control group.

In a recent study conducted by the present authors involving 33 subjects with MS, 10 of whom were dysarthric, significant differences in parameters of intelligibility were identified between the subjects with MS and a control group of normal speakers. Based on the results from the ASSIDS (Yorkston and Beukelman, 1981), the MS group was found to exhibit significant reductions in word intelligibility, rate of speech (words per minute), and communication efficiency (intelligible words per minute/normal rate of 190 words per minute) (see Table 2.4). Although the MS group recorded a slightly lower percentage score for sentence intelligibility compared to the control group, no significant difference between the two groups was obtained for this parameter. The subgroup of dysarthric MS subjects demonstrated a similar pattern of impairment in intelligibility, rate of speech, and communication efficiency to the total MS group. The lack of significant difference in sentence intelligibility between the control group and the dysarthric MS speakers was consistent with the high standard deviation recorded for this parameter, reflecting a wide range of severity of impairment (mild to moderate to severe) in the dysarthric subjects.

Speech subsystem dysfunction in multiple sclerosis

While perceptual rating scales and intelligibility measures have provided descriptions of the speech output in individuals with MS, studies have also been conducted to subjectively investigate the performance of each subsystem of the speech mechanism (respiratory, laryngeal, velopharyngeal, and articulatory) in an attempt to determine the underlying basis of the disordered speech production.

A recent study conducted in our laboratory, in which 30 subjects with MS (10 dysarthrics and 20 non-dysarthrics) were evaluated on the FDA, revealed that the performance of these individuals was significantly different to a matched control group on 23 of the 25 subsystem components of the FDA evaluated. The subjects with MS were found to demonstrate impairments in all subsystems of the speech mechanism except for

Table 2.4 Comparison of the means and standard deviations for the MS group, the dysarthric MS subgroup, and the control group for the intelligibility, rate, and communication efficiency values obtained from the Assessment of Intelligibility of Dysarthric Speech.[1]

Parameter	Total MS group (N=33)		Dysarthric MS group (N=10)		Control group (N=19)	
	M	SD	M	SD	M	SD
% Word Intelligibility	89.87 **	11.82	89.60 **	9.96	99.05	1.54
% Sentence Intelligibility	96.87	10.50	92.72	18.74	99.97	0.11
Words per minute (WPM)	150.94 **	39.54	137.36 *	44.87	187.09	25.59
Communication efficiency ratio (CER)	0.78 **	0.22	0.70 *	0.25	0.98	0.13

** = significant difference compared to control group (p<.001)
* = significant difference compared to control group (p<.01)
[1] = Yorkston & Beukelman (1981)

jaw function. Examination of the level of performance of the subjects with MS on the FDA, however, revealed that overall, subsystem impairment ranged from minimal to mild (see Figure 2.1). Specifically, tongue and laryngeal function were noted to be the most impaired in this group of MS subjects, a finding consistent with the frequent occurrence of articulatory imprecision and dysphonia in MS populations.

When the performance of the 10 dysarthric speakers on the FDA was examined separately, this group was found to demonstrate significant differences to the control group on 23 of the 25 subsystems components. The dysarthric speakers with MS were not observed to demonstrate any impairments in lip and jaw status at rest, compared to the control group. While a similar pattern of dysfunction to the total MS group was observed in the dysarthric speakers, the level of impairment across the subsystems was slightly greater in the latter group, as would be expected considering that the total MS group comprised both dysarthric and non-dysarthric speakers.

In a comparable study, Hartelius et al. (1993), using a series of tasks similar to the FDA, to evaluate respiration, phonation, and oromotor skills (lip, tongue, jaw, soft palate) in a group of 30 Swedish MS subjects, found that these individuals demonstrated significant impairments in each of these aspects of speech production, compared to the control group. A similar finding was evident for the 14 dysarthric MS speakers within this group. Interestingly, Hartelius et al. (1993) found that the dysarthric speakers who were perceived to exhibit a slight to moderate overall speech abnormality tended to demonstrate increasing deficits in respiration, phonation, and oromotor skills that were incommensurate

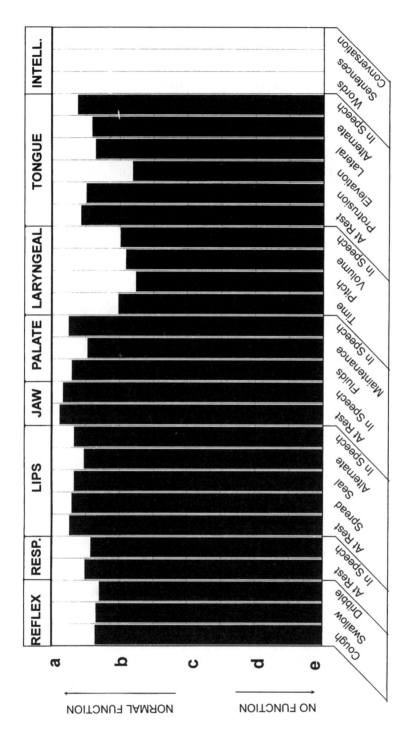

Figure 2.1 Frenchay Dysarthria Profile for 30 subjects with MS

with disturbances in articulation, prosody, and speech intelligibility. On maximum performance measures of expiratory pressure, fricative and vowel durations, oral diadochokinetic rates, and reading rate, the subjects with MS demonstrated a consistently poorer performance on these tasks compared to the control subjects, although these differences were not statistically significant.

It is apparent from both the Australian and Swedish studies of subsystem dysfunction in MS subjects that those with a dysarthric speech disturbance are likely to demonstrate impairment in all subsystems of the speech mechanism. It would appear that impairment in both the laryngeal and articulatory subsystems of the speech mechanism represents the predominant pattern of subsystem dysfunction in these individuals, having been identified in both studies in one form or another. This latter finding is consistent with the high frequency of occurrence of abnormal phonatory and articulatory speech features perceived to be present in the three major studies of MS populations. Although speech subsystem dysfunction has been identified in individuals with MS using relatively subjective perceptual techniques, these findings require confirmation through objective physiological assessment of each of the subsystems of the speech production mechanism.

Subclinical manifestations of motor speech impairment in multiple sclerosis

While the perceptual evaluation of motor speech subsystems in dysarthric speakers with MS has revealed dysfunction in various subsystems, there is evidence to suggest that this form of assessment has the capacity to identify subtle signs of motor speech impairment in the MS population before they manifest clinically as a dysarthric speech disturbance. In the study conducted in our laboratory, while the total MS group and the group of dysarthric speakers were found to be significantly impaired on the majority of components of the FDA, the group of non-dysarthric speakers were also found to demonstrate significant differences in speech subsystem performance, compared to the control group.

In fact, the non-dysarthric MS group were found to be significantly more impaired than the controls on 20 of the 25 components of the FDA. The non-dysarthric speakers exhibited signs of impaired reflex activity in relation to swallowing, coughing, and saliva control, respiratory impairments at rest and during speech, mild lip asymmetry and impairment of lip spread and alternate lip movements, impaired maintenance of palatal movements in isolation and during speech, reduced phonation time, impaired pitch and loudness variability, and abnormal vocal quality. The impairment of tongue function in the non-dysarthric speakers was found to be greater than for lip function in this group, with significant deficits in all non-speech tongue movements (protrusion, elevation, lateral, and alternate) and precision of tongue movements during speech.

Subclinical signs of motor speech dysfunction have also been reported by Hartelius et al. (1993) in their subgroup of 16 non-dysarthric speakers with MS. When assessed on the Hartelius et al. (1993) clinical protocol, the non-dysarthric speakers were found to be significantly more impaired in respiration, phonation, and oromotor skills compared to the control subjects. The greatest differences between the controls and the non-dysarthrics occurred in phonatory and oral musculature function. It would appear from these findings that the laryngeal and articulatory subsystems are perhaps the more vulnerable subsystems with respect to the disease process in MS and are more likely to demonstrate preclinical signs of motor speech impairment. The degree of impairment in the laryngeal subsystem and in tongue function in the non-dysarthric speakers in our study would tend to support this hypothesis. Furthermore, the marked impairment in phonatory and oromotor abilities in the non-dysarthric speakers with MS in the Hartelius et al. (1993) study is consistent with similar findings for dysarthric MS speakers, and the high frequency of occurrence of phonatory and articulatory impairment evident in MS populations.

The subclinical findings of motor speech impairment in persons with MS reported by Hartelius et al. (1993), and also observed in the study conducted by the authors of the present chapter, are consistent with evidence of similar preclinical motor speech dysfunction in other progressive neurologically disordered groups, such as patients with amyotrophic lateral sclerosis (ALS) and patients with Parkinson's disease (PD). Langmore and Lehman (1994) found that non-dysarthric ALS subjects demonstrated physiological decrements in the strength and speed of tongue, lip, and jaw movements. Similarly, De Paul et al. (1988) identified weakness of the tongue, lips, and jaw in their non-dysarthric ALS subjects. As the findings of Hartelius et al. (1993) and those of the current authors are based on subjective measures of motor speech impairment, it is important that the evidence of subclinical manifestations of motor speech impairment in persons with MS in these studies is confirmed, and further investigated, using objective measures of motor speech function such as physiological and acoustic evaluation (see Chapters 3–5).

Summary and conclusions

The dysarthric speech disturbance associated with MS usually presents as a mixed dysarthria, occurring in slightly less than half of the MS population. Initially the speech disorder is mild with the level of severity progressively increasing with greater neurological dysfunction. Persons with MS have been perceived to exhibit abnormal speech features in all aspects of speech production. Specifically, articulatory imprecision, harshness, impaired stress patterns, reduced breath support for speech, and impaired pitch variation are the most prevalent abnormalities in speech production identified in this population. There is evidence to suggest that individuals with MS may demonstrate subclinical features of motor speech impairment prior to the manifestation of a dysarthric speech disturbance. Although perceptual evaluations have identified deviant speech characteristics and clinical and subclinical speech subsystem dysfunction within the MS population, these abnormal features require confirmation, both physiologically and acoustically, before valid and realistic directions for treatment may be determined.

Chapter 3
Acoustic features of dysarthria in multiple sclerosis

Lena Hartelius

Introduction

Acoustic analysis has been used to characterize different aspects of disordered speech for several decades. Increasingly more refined methods of analysis now allow detailed exploration of temporal as well as spectral characteristics of speech. Temporal characteristics are quantifiable through the measurement of duration of different speech events (syllables, speech segments or subsegmental entities such as vowel formant transitions, occlusion or transient phases of stop consonants etc.). Spectral characteristics, on the other hand, are shown by the distribution of energy across the frequency axis (the bandwidth of vowel formants or spectral tilts of fricatives etc.). These temporal and spectral measures assist in describing the articulatory characteristics of speech. Measurements of phonatory characteristics are made by exploring aspects of the glottal waveform, such as frequency of phonatory cycles (fundamental frequency, F_o), cycle-to-cycle variation in pitch period time and amplitude (jitter and shimmer), as well as the relations between periodic and aperiodic energy. These acoustic measures of phonatory characteristics are all thought to reflect perceptual aspects of voice quality. Extracted contours of the frequency and intensity of F_o allow further measurements of mean level and variability (audible as pitch, loudness, monotonicity and stability of these two parameters).

For more detailed information on speech acoustics and its application to the area of dysarthric speech, the reader is referred to Kent and Read (1992) and to recently published chapters such as Farmer (1997), Forrest and Weismer (1997), and Thompson-Ward and Theodoros (1998). The goal of this chapter is to describe efforts that have been made to characterize the dysarthria of multiple sclerosis using acoustic

methods. The first section describes attempts to quantify the characteristic temporal speech disruption mentioned in early descriptions of MS
dysarthria, the so-called 'scanning speech'. The second section is
dedicated to the acoustic correlates of imprecise articulation in multiple
sclerosis and is followed by a section describing phonatory characteristics. The final section illustrates the use of acoustic measures in
monitoring treatment in an individual with multiple sclerosis.

Acoustic analysis of speech in neurological disorders

There are a number of ways in which acoustic analysis of speech and
voice can add to the knowledge of neurological disease:

1. Acoustic analysis provides an interface between speech production
   and perception (Forrest and Weismer, 1997). The acoustic perspective complements the perceptual perspective in identifying and
   quantifying the disordered components of the speech system. The
   acoustic data can also be related to decreases in intelligibility, thereby
   indicating the speech components that are most vulnerable and tend
   to affect the comprehensibility of dysarthric speakers the most (Kent
   et al., 1991).
2. Acoustic analysis can be used to document progressive degeneration
   of motor speech function in certain neurological diseases. This has
   been demonstrated in case studies of individuals with amyotrophic
   lateral sclerosis (ALS) by Ramig et al. (1990) and Kent et al. (1991).
   Ramig et al. (1990) measured different aspects of sustained phonation and observed increasing phonatory instability and reduced
   phonatory limits over a time period of six months. Kent et al. (1991)
   documented a decline in the average slope of the second formant
   frequency which was paralleled by a successive reduction in intelligibility over a two-year period, indicating progressive loss of lingual
   control. Because acoustic analysis can be used to document progressive degeneration, it also has the potential of documenting recovery
   or effects of treatment.
3. Acoustic analysis may identify subclinical manifestations of neurological disease. That is, nascent disease symptoms might reveal
   themselves in selected acoustic measures in the absence of dysarthric
   signs in continuous speech. Ramig, Titze et al. (1988) compared
   subjects with Huntington's disease (HD) to subjects at risk for HD
   and to normal controls. They found the incidence of the low
   frequency segments (abrupt drops in frequency of approximately one
   octave) characteristic of the phonation in individuals with HD to be

12 times as great in the subjects at risk for HD as that observed in the normal control group. All subjects at risk for HD were judged by a speech pathologist as having perceptually normal voices.

Multiple sclerosis is also a chronic illness partly characterized by subclinical disease activity and there have been a few attempts over the years to use acoustic analyses to detect early diagnostic signs of the illness (Scripture, 1916, 1933; Zemlin, 1962; Haggard, 1969; Hartelius, Buder and Strand, 1997). These studies focused on the detection of irregularities in sustained phonation and will be described in more detail below. The sporadic interest in phonatory irregularities in multiple sclerosis indicates that we might be going around in circles, and the only thing that differentiates the MS phonation researcher today from the one in 1916 is the power of the tools. The question is still not completely investigated, but with the increasing development and availability of acoustic methods we are increasingly better equipped for more refined analyses.

4. Acoustic analysis may contribute to differential diagnosis by elucidating the involvement of different neural subsystems. Combinations of dysarthric symptoms may reflect different underlying pathophysiologies, for instance, weakness, spasticity, ataxia, or tremor. These signs of underlying pathophysiologies are indicative of site of lesion in the nervous system, and if they can be independently quantified, they can be used in differential diagnosis. Ramig, Titze et al. (1988) demonstrated distinct systematic differences in vocal patterns for patients with myotonic dystrophy (large cycle-to-cycle disruptions in amplitude and frequency, i.e. shimmer and jitter), Huntington's disease (abrupt phonatory disruptions indicating choreatic movement jerks), and Parkinson's disease (long-term phonatory instability in the form of amplitude tremor). Furthermore, there is an interesting speculation concerning vocal tremor that warrants further investigation. Winholz and Ramig (1992) put forward the idea that the amplitude or magnitude (i.e. the extent of the tremulous oscillatory movement) could be related to the extent or progression of neurological disorder and that the frequency of tremor (i.e. the rate of the oscillatory movement) could suggest involvement of a particular neural subsystem. However, there is considerable overlap among the tremor frequency ranges associated with different neurological disorders as well as between normal and some pathological tremor frequencies, although pathological tremor generally is considered to be slower than normal physiological tremor. Three studies of cerebellar ataxic tremor have identified a phonatory tremor frequency range of 1.5–3 Hz (Ackerman and Ziegler, 1991; Ackerman and Ziegler, 1994; Hartelius et al., 1995).

Modern techniques of acoustic speech analysis allow virtually every aspect of speech to be measured. Hence, it is of great importance to identify those aspects which can tell us something important about the speech disorder, that is to establish their clinical validity. What is to be considered normal or pathological is not always a clearcut issue. There is considerable individual variability on different acoustic measures. Acoustic manifestations of dysarthric signs like inadequate closure or voicing during voiceless stop consonants, shallow slopes of formant two transitions etc. can all be found to some degree in normal speech as well, at least in the more reduced 'hypospeech' forms. Whether we judge the speech to be normal or pathological could be a matter of severity of signs or a matter of number of signs during a given unit of time. In our search for valid and reliable information about dysarthria, we should always combine acoustic measures with the corresponding perceptual impressions and, to ensure clinical validity, with as detailed information as possible about the dysarthric speaker's underlying neuropathology.

The perceptual speech characteristics of multiple sclerosis are described in detail in Chapter 2 of this book. The type of dysarthria associated with multiple sclerosis has been described as a 'mixed spastic-ataxic dysarthria'. The spastic characteristics (determined by lesions of the corticobulbar tracts) are thought to be defective articulation, hyper-nasality, variable pitch, breathiness, and harshness. The ataxic character-istics (determined by cerebellar lesions) are thought to be impaired loudness control, defective articulation, and 'scanning speech' (Griffiths and Bough, 1989). These symptoms are shared by other types of dysarthria as well, notably spastic and ataxic dysarthria. Hence, it is not possible at this stage to find the typical acoustic manifestation of MS dysarthria. We can only use our instrumental tools to quantify relevant aspects of this complex type of dysarthria. The aspects focused on here are mainly 'scanning speech', imprecise articulation and phonatory characteristics. The questions asked are: (a) How can the timing difficul-ties of certain speakers with multiple sclerosis be explained and quanti-fied with acoustic measures?, (b) Are there specific articulatory features typical of individuals with multiple sclerosis that can be acoustically displayed?, (c) Do subclinical speech signs exist, e.g. in sustained phona-tion, and can they be quantified with acoustic measures?, and, finally (d) How can acoustic analysis assist in treatment decisions regarding individuals with multiple sclerosis?

'Scanning speech' in multiple sclerosis

'Scanning speech' was one of the three cardinal symptoms of multiple sclerosis described by Charcot (1877). His description of this characteristic has frequently been cited in its English translation: 'The words are as if measured or scanned; there is a pause after every syllable, and the syllables themselves are pronounced slowly.' Scripture (1916) strongly argued against the use of this term, and stated that:

> The term 'scanning' is applied in prosody to marking off the long and short or the loud and weak syllables, that is, to indicate the maxima and minima. In scanning a line of verse with the voice, the speaker exaggerates the differences between the two kinds of syllables, making the emphatic syllables more emphatic (longer or louder) and the unemphatic ones less marked (shorter or weaker). This is exactly what the patient with disseminated sclerosis does not do.

He continued the description of what the speaker with multiple sclerosis does not do and finally concluded:

> We are justified in concluding that the speech, as far as the durations are concerned, simply shares in the general ataxia and spasticity and that its peculiarities are the results of ataxia and spasticity and the efforts to control them. The term 'scanning speech' cannot be used.

In spite of this compelling argument, 'scanning speech' has in the meantime become one of the most frequently used terms in the characterization of MS dysarthria. Not all dysarthric individuals with multiple sclerosis have a predominantly ataxic dysarthria, but the 'scanning' characteristic is shared also by dysarthric individuals with cerebellar lesions of different aetiologies and has consequently been used in the characterization of purely ataxic dysarthria as well. Brown et al. (1970) used the term 'excess and equal stress' as an equivalent perceptual term and defined it as a disorder of prosody where excess vocal emphasis is placed on usually unstressed syllables and words. Several efforts have been made to quantify this characteristic in ataxic dysarthria with acoustic measures. The most common findings have been lengthened and equalized syllable durations (Kent et al., 1975; Kent et al., 1979; Ackerman and Hertrich, 1993). A seemingly contradictory temporal characteristic has also been noted, namely an increased variability of syllable as well as segment durations (Ackerman and Hertrich, 1993; Kent et al., 1997). Ackerman and Hertrich (1993) noted a tendency towards syllable equalization within sentences but also a simultaneous tendency towards increased variability in syllable duration in repetitions of the same sentence.

To summarize, there are several studies showing that the acoustic correlate of 'scanning speech' or 'excess and equal stress' is equalization of syllable durations. The studies have so far only included individuals with purely ataxic dysarthria, not with MS dysarthria. However, there are indications that this characteristic is emanating from the cerebellar component in the speech disorder. According to FitzGerald et al. (1987), all of their MS subjects with deviations in stress had some degree of cerebellar dysfunction. At the syllabic level, what is expected from the normal speaker is variability, that is, differences in syllable durations in consecutive strings of syllables. What the individual with 'scanning speech' does, however, is to produce syllable durations that are isochronous, 'at equal time'. However, there are other units of speech, where isochrony is indeed expected from the normal speaker.

The stress group is such a unit, consisting of one stressed and several unstressed syllables. The stress groups are supposed to be initiated at regular absolute time intervals measurable as interstress interval durations, the beginning of each group coinciding with the onset of the vowel in the stressed syllable (Lehiste, 1977; Eriksson, 1991). These time intervals are thought to be kept regular despite variability in the various subcomponents of the syllables (Keller, 1990). In order to investigate the temporal characteristics of individuals with multiple sclerosis and ataxic dysarthria, Hartelius et al. (2000) explored the following questions: (a) at the syllabic level, are individuals with multiple sclerosis and ataxic dysarthria more isochronic than variable, that is do they exhibit syllable equalization? (b) is the assumed isochrony different comparing syllable lengths intra-utterance (within the same sentence) versus inter-utterance (in repetitions of the same sentence)? (c) at the interstress interval level, where we expect isochrony, are these individuals able to perform this intended isochrony or are they in fact more variable than matched normal controls?

The subjects selected for study by Hartelius et al. (2000) were selected from a larger MS population of 77 individuals, studied by Hartelius et al. (1999, 2000). Fourteen subjects with predominantly ataxic dysarthria were selected for this study, using the following procedure. Two independent speech clinicians, experienced in the assessment of dysarthric speech, made perceptual judgements of all 77 MS individuals as well as 15 control subjects. These judgements were made on randomized recorded samples of text reading. Judgements included ratings of the 32 perceptual dimensions adapted from Darley et al. (1969a, b) and used in FitzGerald et al. (1987). Mean intrarater reliability was calculated using Spearman Rank Order Correlation and found to be rho 0.80 while mean interrater reliability was 0.69. The judges also made an overall assessment of severity of speech deviation and rated to what degree the speech of each individual was perceived as being predominantly ataxic, spastic, flaccid, and hypokinetic, respectively. For the present study, the 14 subjects with the highest scores on ataxic dysarthria from both judges were selected. Seven of these individuals were judged by a neurologist as having a substantial cerebellar involvement (operationally defined as a score of ≥ 3 on the cerebellar functional system according to Kurtzke's scoring system (Kurtzke, 1983b).

Syllable durations and durations of interstress intervals were measured for each individual in five different sentences, each repeated three times. Mean durations and coefficients of variation (the standard deviations divided by their respective means) were used to illustrate level and variability of temporal control in these subjects. Referring to our initial questions, the following conclusions can be drawn:

(a) At the syllable level, we found that the MS group showed significantly *increased syllable durations* compared to the control group. The MS group was also significantly less variable (more isochronous) in the performance of consecutive syllable production within a sentence.

(b) The MS group showed significantly *decreased intra-utterance variability* but at the same time *increased inter-utterance variability* compared to the control group, as measured by the coefficient of variation in syllable duration.

(c) At the interstress interval level significantly *increased durations* in the MS group compared to the control group were found. At this level we also found a statistically significantly *increased variability (less isochrony)* compared to the control group, contrary to what was expected.

The results of this study clearly show that temporal dysregulation is indeed a primary characteristic of ataxic dysarthria in MS. This is well in agreement with the findings of other recent studies of ataxic dysarthria (Ackerman and Hertrich, 1993; Ziegler et al., 1993; Kent et al., 1997). The contradictory tendencies towards syllable equalization within sentences on the one hand and syllable duration variability between sentences on the other hand, identified by Ackerman and Hertrich (1993) were also found in this study. Hence, the temporal dysregulation associated with ataxic dysarthria and MS has been confirmed. However, the perceptual correlate to this temporal dysregulation, the audible signs of 'scanning speech' might not be the syllable equalization. The results of this study point to the possibility of the interstress interval being another important entity, where the lack of even rhythmic beats (even interstress intervals) could contribute to the audible dysrhythmic character of ataxic dysarthria.

As also found by Ackerman and Hertrich (1993), the tendency towards variability was stronger than the one towards isochrony. The tendency towards syllable equalization within sentences could be a reflection of an inability to shorten syllables when appropriate, this inability being primarily founded in articulatory constraints. This would mean that the syllable equalization is not primarily a dysprosodic characteristic, but a feature secondary to the articulatory deficiencies.

The inconsistency in the perceptual impressions of ataxic dysarthria has been discussed earlier, for example by Kent et al. (1997), and it has been suggested that this inconsistency may be resolved by using quantitative acoustic analysis. The results reported in the study described here suggest that the inconsistency is in fact present in the acoustic signal and forms a part of the characteristics of the speech of individuals with cerebellar involvement. It could be true both that limited variability is a primary characteristic of these individuals and that this is audible as prosodic insufficiency and measurable in the acoustic signal as syllable equalization and an inflexibility in changing speaking rate. This is thought to be caused by inflexibility in temporal control. On the other hand it could also be true that increased variability is a primary characteristic, audible as prosodic excess and measurable as increased variability across repetitions of the same sentence as well as variability in duration of interstress intervals, this being a reflection of instability of temporal control. Syllable equalization, a possible sign of prosodic insufficiency, did in fact exist together with uneven interstress intervals, a possible sign of prosodic excess in some of the individuals investigated in this study.

Imprecise Articulation in Multiple Sclerosis

FitzGerald et al. (1987) found imprecise consonants and distorted vowels to be comparatively frequent in the speech of their MS subjects (in 83% and 57% respectively). Acoustic measurements of defective articulation have generally involved measures of second formant (F2) movements in consonant-vowel transitions, as the extent and duration of the F2 transition have been found to correlate to speech intelligibility (Kent et al., 1991). So far, acoustic data describing the articulatory characteristics of individuals with multiple sclerosis have been very scarce and more qualitative than quantitative in nature. Hartelius et al. (1995) provided examples of various articulatory features evident in the acoustic signal of five speakers with multiple sclerosis, most of which were general manifestations of imprecise consonants also compatible with other types of dysarthria. Among the features exemplified were spirantization (continuous frication caused by inadequate closure), continuous voicing during voiceless consonants, nasal formant during voiced plosives, and instability of the voicing onset following stop releases. Although not quantified, the F2 movements in the speech of the individuals with multiple sclerosis were frequently found to be slower (having longer transition durations), more shallow (having reduced transition extents), and to extend over more than 50% of the total vowel duration, thereby indicating inertia of the tongue musculature. The instability of the voicing onset following stop releases was also found by Sanderson et al. (1996) who investigated a group of eight individuals with multiple sclerosis. In their study, this characteristic is described as multiple consonant release bursts in voiced and voiceless plosives.

Efforts are also being made to quantify articulatory changes during bouts of the illness in individuals with multiple sclerosis (Seikel et al., 1996). Connected speech and sustained vowel phonations of four subjects with multiple sclerosis have been analysed pre-, peri-, and post exacerbation. Although the intersubject variability was substantial, results point to decreased segment durations as well as decreased formant values during, as compared to pre- and post exacerbation.

The acoustic measurement of dysarthric articulation is an area that needs further exploration. A methodology is needed that can reliably quantify the changes made in the energy distribution across the frequency range over time, to reflect not only the restricted range in articulatory movements but also the lack of contrasts over time. These characteristics also need to be related to intelligibility and speech rate. Buder et al. (1996) described a method of analysis of spectral characteristics that can be displayed in temporal succession. This technique may prove very useful in describing these characteristics.

Phonatory characteristics of dysarthria in multiple sclerosis

According to previous studies, the three most common perceptual signs of MS dysarthria are phonatory ones: impaired loudness control, tremulous pitch and harsh voice quality (Darley et al., 1972; FitzGerald et al., 1987). Underlying all efforts to characterize MS phonation with acoustic methods have been the intriguing questions of whether phonatory irregularities exist independently of a manifest speech disorder, and if they can be detected as early diagnostic or subclinical signs of the illness.

Efforts to use short-term acoustic measures of phonatory dysfunction (cycle-to-cycle variations in frequency and amplitude, i.e. measures of jitter and shimmer) have not proven very successful in discriminating dysarthric from nondysarthric individuals. Long-term acoustic measures, on the other hand, have been used to quantify the slower, cyclic variation in frequency and intensity occurring at frequencies lower than the glottal cycle. These measures are more suitable for describing the long-term phonatory instabilities associated with neurological laryngeal pathologies, for example tremor (Zwirner et al., 1991; Kent et al., 1994). Apart from visual inspection of the waveform or oscillogram as a qualitative index of tremor, long-term phonatory instabilities have so far been measured mainly in two different ways.

First as the coefficients of variation for both amplitude and frequency (the standard deviations of the amplitude and frequency during sustained phonation divided by their respective means). Secondly, spectrum analysis (or Fast Fourier Transform, FFT) has been used to obtain measures of the magnitude and rate of tremor oscillations in both frequency and intensity during sustained phonation. This technique can go beyond the overall measure of extent or amplitude of the instability, enabling us to see whether the instability is periodic or not, and if so, which frequency components contribute to the instability.

In describing the phonatory irregularities associated with multiple sclerosis, both short-term and long-term measurements have been used. Scripture (1916, 1933) used what seemed to be a kymograph and noted 'small, irregular waves' (pressure variations) in the sustained vowel phonations of all of his 20 MS subjects, which included both dysarthric and nondysarthric individuals. These waves were most prominent in the beginning and towards the end of phonation and were explained as instances of laryngeal ataxia. Zemlin (1962) measured periodicity in vocal fold vibration and found significant differences between the 33 individuals with multiple sclerosis and the normal controls. Zemlin (1962) also noted that a subgroup of his subjects exhibited a predictable, cyclic period change, more prominent on /a/ than on /i/ phonation. The recordings of 26 nondysarthric individuals with multiple sclerosis were studied by Haggard (1969). He too observed both amplitude and frequency phonatory variability from cycle to cycle. However, both Zemlin (1962) and Haggard (1969) identified individuals with completely normal phonatory patterns among their subjects with multiple sclerosis.

Preliminary data using FFT analysis in describing the phonation of five individuals with multiple sclerosis and two control speakers (Hartelius et al., 1995) showed that many of the instabilities produced by the subjects with multiple sclerosis were greater in both magnitude and frequency than those produced by the control subjects. The individuals with multiple sclerosis differed in their spectrum peak locations (i.e. predominant tremor frequencies), but the instabilities occurred within a 1–4 Hz frequency band and the individual speakers seemed to be fairly consistent across different vowels. A prominent 3 Hz tremor was found in a male MS subject who had cerebellar ataxia and a small, but clearly discernible 4 Hz tremor was found in a female MS subject who had no audible dysarthric symptoms.

Encouraged by these preliminary results, and with the primary purpose of providing a more comprehensive description and quantification of long-term phonatory instability in an MS population, a larger investigation was carried out (Hartelius, Buder and Strand, 1997). The study included 20 individuals with a definite diagnosis of multiple sclerosis and 20 age- and gender-matched control subjects (with a mean age of 44 years, and with 9 males and 11 females in each group).

The subjects with multiple sclerosis represented varying stages of disease progression and mean time post diagnosis was 7.6 years. Fourteen individuals with multiple sclerosis (70%) were nondysarthric, while six (30%) had varying degrees of dysarthria, as rated by five experienced judges. All subjects were recorded sustaining the vowels /a/, /i/, and /u/ for as long as possible at a comfortable frequency and intensity level. In the first step of analysis the sustained vowel phonations were digitized and fundamental frequency (F_o) and intensity (dB) contours were extracted. In the second step the last 2.5 seconds of each F_o and dB contours were converted into time-series data and subjected to Fourier (spectral) analysis. This part of the phonation was selected to ensure comparability across individual samples and because tremor was typically (but not always) observed towards the end of phonation. The magnitudes and frequencies of spectral peaks were then identified as correlates of tremor, and different statistical methods of analysis were used to explore the data. The methods of analysis are described in detail in Hartelius, Buder and Strand (1997).

The results of the study were as follows:

1. Statistically significant differences between subjects with multiple sclerosis and the matched group of control subjects were found on all measures of long-term phonatory instability. This was true for both acoustic intensity and fundamental frequency parameters, with the largest significant differences between MS and normal controls being observed in the intensity parameter. Age was found to be correlated to the F_o related measures only in the normal group. There were no significant differences in levels of instability between men and women in either group as measured by any of the variables. In comparing different vowels, the order of observed instability was similar within both groups: /a/ > /i/ > /u/.

2. These differences remained even between nondysarthric subjects with multiple sclerosis and their controls. This points to the existence of subclinical speech symptoms. Subjects with multiple sclerosis often report that speech production is 'different' or demands more

energy, even while the motor speech system is apparently still able to compensate for the impairment. The acoustic measures used in this study demonstrated a sensitivity to these subclinical signs. While some may argue that phonatory differences which are not yet perceptually evident have no clinical validity or importance, identification of these subclinical signs may allow clinicians to predict more accurately which patients are likely to develop increasing laryngeal involvement as well as dysarthria. This could lead to better timing of early intervention. In addition, the ability to reliably detect phonatory changes (that may not be easily measured perceptually) may be very useful in measuring results of pharmacological treatment in many neurological diseases.

3. Individuals with multiple sclerosis exhibited different patterns of magnitudes and frequencies of instability in F_o and intensity, and these differences were repeatable across successive phonations by the same subjects. The individual patterns may be systematically related to different neuropathologies and/or subsystem impairments. However, the lack of sufficiently detailed neurologic data on the patients included in this particular MS population prevented further exploration of the relationship between phonatory patterns and specific neuropathology.

In conclusion, it is possible to detect and to differentiate individual patterns of long-term phonatory instability in individuals with multiple sclerosis even in those individuals who do not exhibit any perceptually evident dysarthria or laryngeal involvement.

The use of acoustic analysis in monitoring treatment variables in individuals with multiple sclerosis: a case study

There is increasing evidence supporting the benefit of speech therapy for different groups of dysarthric speakers (for recent review of interventions suited for different dysarthria types, see Yorkston et al., 1988; McNeil, 1997). However, so far extremely few studies have focused on the improvement of speech in individuals with multiple sclerosis. Farmakides and Boone (1960) showed that 85% of the 68 treated MS patients improved their speech as a result of the speech training. The success of therapy was explained as a reduction of disuse atrophy in affected musculature. In addition, in a treatment study to investigate the use of visual feedback to enhance prosodic control, one of three subjects included had MS (Caligiuri and Murry, 1983). This subject not only showed improvements in speaking rate, prosodic control and a reduction in

overall severity, but he also demonstrated an improvement in articulatory precision, thought to be secondary to the gains associated with
reduction in speaking rate and increased prosodic control. The use of
acoustic analysis in monitoring dysarthria treatment has been
documented earlier in studies of ataxic dysarthria by Berry and Goshorn
(1983), Caligiuri and Murry (1983) and Simmons (1983), and in a study
of hypokinetic dysarthria by Adams (1994). Subsequently, the attempts
to use acoustic analyses to document possible treatment effects in
dysarthria have been few, and in the case of individuals with multiple
sclerosis almost non-existent. The case described below is drawn from a
study of seven individuals with multiple sclerosis that participated in a
recent speech intervention programme (Hartelius, Wising and Nord,
1997).

Case presentation

EB is a 36-year-old woman diagnosed with multiple sclerosis four years
prior to assessment. She was referred to the speech clinic by her neurologist on her own request because she had problems articulating; she
found her speech to be 'thicker' and 'more effortful'. The neurologist
did not find any of these symptoms to be particularly prominent, but
recognized her need to be evaluated and counselled by a speech pathologist. She was still in a relapsing-remitting stage of her disease with a
disability score of 6.5 (on Kurtzke's (1983b) Expanded Disability Status
Scale – EDSS – from 0 to 10) and she was walking with support. Her
speech problem was assessed by the speech clinician to be of a mild
cerebellar type with uncoordinated speech breathing, uncontrolled
variations in loudness and pitch, and harsh voice quality. She was also
judged to have a slight hypernasality and weakness and inco-ordination
in her oral musculature manifested in a slow and dysrhythmic diado-
chokinesis. These signs were most apparent in a systematic evaluation of
the respiratory, phonatory and oral motor systems. In connected speech,
she was able to compensate fairly well using a somewhat reduced
speech rate. However, the slowed speech carried signs of excess and
equal stress.

EB was invited to participate in 14 training sessions (4 individual
sessions and 10 in a group consisting of patients with multiple sclerosis
and similar speech problems). Briefly, the training programme had three
objectives; (a) increased vocal efficiency, (b) effective use of contrastive
stress, and (c) effective use of verbal repair strategies.[1] After the interven-

---

[1] The reader is referred to Hartelius, Wising and Nord (1997) for a more detailed
description of the rationale for and the outline of the intervention programme.

tion period, three sets of speech samples were perceptually evaluated pairwise in a randomized order (pre- and post-therapy) by independent judges: (a) passage reading, (b) contrastive stress sentences, and (c) four versions of the same sentence; one uncorrected and one repaired version (the patient was requested to repeat a particular sentence 'to make it easier to understand'), pre- as well as post-therapy. The recordings were also analysed acoustically to explore the physical correlates of these perceptual judgements.

Passage reading

Results of the perceptual evaluation showed that EB's post-therapy passage reading was clearly superior to the pre-therapy reading regarding 'articulatory precision' and 'voice' (i.e. F_o and intensity level and variability). However, the third parameter, 'naturalness', was judged to be superior only to a slight degree. It should be mentioned that during the intervention period, EB had three additional bouts of the illness (one bulbar and two incidences of optic neuritis), making it less likely that the changes in her speech could be explained by a coinciding remission period, or any other known medical events.

Contrastive stress sentences

EB could reliably signal contrastive stress pre- as well as post-therapy, that is, the word that EB intended to stress was also the word perceived as stressed by the judges in more than 90% of the instances, both before and after therapy. However, acoustic analysis of these sentences added valuable information to the perceptual analysis. Figure 3.1 (a–d) depicts how she varied her fundamental frequency to achieve this prominence. The sentence is 'Bussens förare fick körkortet indraget' ('The bus driver's licence was revoked') with the stress location placed on four different words in the sentence. (These measures were taken using the Kay Elemetrics Computerized Speech Lab, model 4300B). Although the stressed word has a higher fundamental frequency than surrounding unstressed words both pre- and post-therapy, the peak F_o in the stressed word is higher post- than pre-therapy and there is a greater range of F_o variability post-therapy, which could not be reliably detected by the ear. These acoustic measures can be interpreted as an indication of existing degrees of freedom; a phonatory 'working space' which could be expanded to counteract further limitations in the future as the disease progresses.

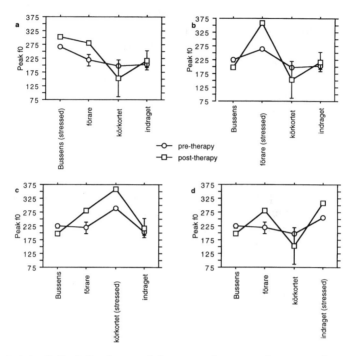

Figure 3.1 (a–d) Peak fundamental frequency in stressed compared to unstressed words pre- and post-therapy. Error bars = ± 1 standard error.

Verbal repairs

Spectrograms (using a KAY DSP 5500 work station) of a part of the sentence used for verbal repair analysis are shown in Figure 3.2. The sentence begins 'Men då kan han ...' ('In that case couldn't he ...') and two versions of the sentence are compared for EB; the uncorrected version pre-therapy and the repaired version post-therapy. Several things are worth noticing in the post-therapy repaired version, mainly that she is slowing her speech rate in response to the request for a verbal repair, allowing for smoother, more elaborate articulatory movements (the cursors are enclosing the transition phase in the syllable [do:], with a clear formant two movements in the repaired sentence). The continuous frication overlaying this part of the sentence is no longer present in the repaired version indicating a more forceful articulation and/or reduction in hypernasality and breathiness of phonation. Particularly prominent is the difference in the articulation of the [k]; in the pre-therapy version there is no complete occlusion (and it is perceptually perceived more as a velar voiced fricative), while the post-therapy version shows a firm occlusion with a distinct release transient phase before the following vowel.

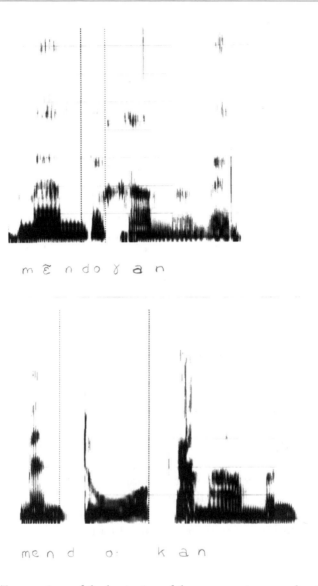

Figure 3.2 Two versions of the beginning of the same sentence spoken by EB; top spectrogram uncorrected version pre-therapy, lower spectrogram corrected version post-therapy.

These examples show how the exploration of EB's speech and her treatment outcome in both perceptual and acoustic terms assisted in characterizing her speech problem and in determining which variables could change. Although it was not tried in this case, spectrographic analysis could easily have been used as a visual feedback tool for EB in her efforts to modify her own speech.

Conclusions

Referring to the questions stated in the introductory section and based on the acoustic studies of MS dysarthria reviewed in this chapter, the following very tentative conclusions can be made: Temporal dysregulation of speech events seems indeed to be a primary characteristic of MS dysarthria. However, equalization of syllable duration might not be the only acoustic correlate to the perceived dysprosody or timing deficiency. The interstress interval could be another important entity, where the lack of even rhythmic beats could also contribute to the audible dysrhythmic character of this type of dysarthria. The tendency towards temporal variability seems to be stronger than the one towards temporal equalization, and it is conceivable that the latter is an effect of articulatory difficulties.

The articulatory characteristics of MS dysarthria include features common to many types of dysarthria and this is an area of research that needs to be expanded further. Interpretation of articulatory acoustic data might also be successfully complemented by simultaneous physiological registration of speech movements. Subclinical speech signs in individuals with multiple sclerosis do exist, and can be documented both as increased fluctuations in sustained phonation and also as increased variability of temporal control. Acoustic analysis provides an excellent tool for reliably detecting such signs. Acoustic analysis can also assist in documenting the range of performance of MS subjects on different speech variables (such as variability of loudness and fundamental frequency, possibility of varying speech rate and articulatory precision). Such information will enable the clinician to tailor intervention procedures for individual patients. Acoustic analysis used in the identification of subclinical speech signs might not be primarily important for early diagnosis of the disease, but for identification of future dysarthric speakers. In addition, it has its main potential as a reliable measure of illness progression and also in a future role as an outcome measure in clinical pharmacological trials.

Chapter 4
Articulatory and velopharyngeal dysfunction in multiple sclerosis

BRUCE E MURDOCH, DEBORAH G THEODOROS AND
ELIZABETH C WARD

Introduction

As indicated in the previous chapter, dysarthria is a common finding in persons with multiple sclerosis (MS). Reports in the literature have indicated that dysarthria may occur in up to 44% of persons with MS (Darley et al., 1972; FitzGerald et al., 1987; Hartelius and Svensson, 1994). Despite the relatively high incidence of dysarthria in MS, however, there is a paucity of research into the specific nature of the motor speech impairment associated with this condition. Speech characteristics of the dysarthria manifested by persons with MS include, among others, articulatory imprecision, nasal voice quality, weak phonation, harshness, breathiness, decreased pitch variability, impaired respiratory support for speech and slow rate. Consequently, it would appear that all aspects of speech production can be disturbed in MS including articulation, resonance, phonation, respiration and prosody. Based on studies of the speech disorders present in other groups of neurologically impaired persons (e.g. Parkinson's disease), it is known that the clinical presentation of dysarthria may result from impairments in the movement and synchrony of the components of the speech production mechanism in terms of range, timing, force, speed or direction (Abbs and De Paul, 1989). However, the way in which these neuromuscular impairments lead to dysarthria in MS remains poorly understood. In particular, the physiological basis of dysarthria in MS has to date received little attention from researchers.

The present chapter reviews previous and current research into the nature and severity of articulatory and velopharyngeal dysfunction in MS, with particular emphasis given to the findings of recently completed

research that has utilized a range of specialized instruments to investigate the physiological functioning of the articulatory and velopharyngeal
components of the speech production mechanism in speakers with MS.
A review of the literature relating to laryngeal and respiratory dysfunction in MS is presented in Chapter 5.

Articulatory dysfunction in multiple sclerosis

Perceptual features of articulatory dysfunction in multiple sclerosis

Studies based on perceptual analyses of the speech disturbance in MS
have provided evidence that dysfunction of the articulatory subsystem
plays a major role in contributing to the reduced speech intelligibility
observed in these cases (Farmakides and Boone, 1960; Darley et al.,
1972; FitzGerald et al., 1987; Hartelius et al., 1993). Defective articulation was present in 46% of the subjects with MS studied by Darley et al.
(1972), and Farmakides and Boone (1960) noted that in many MS
patients with dysarthria 'the movements of the tongue become so slow,
sluggish and weak that articulation becomes slurred and indistinct' (p.
386). Imprecision of consonant production was the most common articulatory deficit encountered in the speech of the patients with MS
examined by FitzGerald et al. (1987), occurring in 83% of their subjects.
Further, imprecision of consonant production was noted by these
workers to be the speech deviation which had the greatest contribution
to variations in overall intelligibility of speech of MS speakers. Recently,
the authors of the present chapter examined a further pool of 33 MS
cases using the same perceptual analysis as used by Fitzgerald et al.
(1987). When combined with the 23 cases investigated by the latter
researchers, 52% of the total 56 cases were found to exhibit deviant
speech dimensions associated with defective articulation.

Physiological assessment of articulation in multiple sclerosis

A variety of different instrumental techniques have been developed to
assess the functioning of the lips, tongue and jaw, many of which have
the potential to be used to determine the articulatory abilities of
speakers with MS. Of the various types of instruments used to assess the
articulators, the most frequently employed to record movement and
force generating capacities of the lips, tongue and jaw have been those
based on strain-gauge transducers. Due to their high levels of sensitivity,
strain-gauge transducers are especially suited to detecting the subtle
changes in movement that occur during speech production. They also
have the advantage of being relatively inexpensive, non-invasive, provide

an immediate voltage analogue of movement and can be adapted to assess lip, tongue and jaw function during both speech and non-speech tasks. Strain-gauge transduction systems have been used by a number of researchers to assess the force generating capacities and the force control capabilities of the lips, tongue and jaw (Barlow and Abbs, 1983; Barlow and Netsell, 1986; McNeil et al., 1990; Langmore and Lehman, 1994; McHenry et al., 1994; Theodoros et al., 1995; Thompson et al., 1995a). In the majority of cases, the basic configuration of the strain-gauge transduction systems used by these authors involved the mounting of strain-gauges (variable resistors) on either side of a flexible metal strip that was anchored at one end to a stable support to form a cantilever. The free end of the cantilever could then be moved by a force produced by either the lips, tongue or jaw.

In addition to strain-gauge transducers, valuable information regarding the functioning of the articulators can be gained from pressure or force transducers. A miniature semi-conductor pressure transducer for measuring interlabial contact pressures during speech was recently trialled by Hinton and Luschei (1992). Due to its small size, this pressure transducer allows for the accurate measurement of the pressures generated between the lips during speech production without interfering with normal articulatory movements. More recently, Thompson-Ward et al. (1999) have interfaced this type of pressure transducer with a dedicated software package to allow for investigations of combined lip pressures, pressure control, endurance and bilabial speech pressures in normal and dysarthric speakers. Pressure transducers have also been used to examine the strength and endurance of the tongue. Robin et al. (1991, 1992) used the Iowa Oral Performance Instrument (IOPI) to examine tongue strength and endurance in normal and articulation disordered persons. This instrument, comprising a 1ml rubber bulb attached to a pressure transducer, is placed in the mouth and the subject instructed to squeeze the bulb against the hard palate with the tongue. An instrument based on the IOPI has been used by Theodoros et al. (1995) and Thompson et al. (1995b) to examine tongue function in a variety of dysarthric speakers and would be suitable for use with persons with MS.

Another popular technique that has been used to examine the functioning of the lips, tongue and jaw is electromyography (EMG) (Folkins and Abbs, 1975; Barlow and Burton, 1988; Shaiman, 1989). Using this technique, the momentary changes in electrical activity that occur when a muscle is contracting are recorded by using either surface electrodes, needle electrodes or hook-wire electrodes. EMG has the potential to be used to investigate the presence of hypertonicity or abnormal variations in the activation and inhibition of activity in the articulatory musculature of speakers with MS.

The location and timing of tongue contacts with the hard palate during speech can be examined by electropalatography. This technique involves the patient wearing an acrylic palate fitted with an array of contact sensors implanted on the surface (Hardcastle et al., 1985). The contact patterns are displayed on a microcomputer. Unfortunately, the use of electropalatography as a routine clinical tool is limited by the need for individual acrylic palates to be constructed for each patient, which is both time-consuming and expensive. However, the technique does offer considerable potential as a research tool for gaining further insight into the physiological basis of tongue dysfunction in MS.

Evaluating the movements of the tongue is more difficult than assessing lip or jaw movement due to the location of the tongue in the oral cavity, with only the anterior section directly observable. Further, the complex muscular arrangement of the tongue allows an almost infinite combination of movements, which can occur at a very rapid rate. For these reasons techniques that generate high resolution movement data are required to examine the dynamics of lingual function. Until recently the principal techniques available and capable of generating such data have included cineradiography and an x-ray microbeam system, both of which are based on x-ray technology. Cineradiography is a high-speed x-ray motion picture technique, which records the lateral view of the pharyngo-oro-nasal complex (Kent et al., 1975). The method allows for the observations and quantification of a number of vocal tract parameters without significantly interfering with normal articulation. Several researchers have used cineradiography in combination with small radio-opaque markers (lead pellets) attached to the articulatory surfaces with biomedical adhesive. This type of assessment allows for examination of the range, velocity and consistency of the movement of the articulators as well as the degree of coordination of the articulators (Hirose et al., 1978).

The major limitation of cineradiography for the assessment of articulatory function is the need to expose the patient to radiation during the procedure. The issue of radiation exposure, however, has been addressed to some extent by introduction of the x-ray microbeam technique (Hirose et al., 1978). The use of this system has greatly reduced the radiation dosage and in conjunction with the use of lead pellets to track and record articulatory movements has increased the advantages of cineradiographic techniques. However, the fact that the system is expensive and still requires some radiation exposure limits the clinical application of this procedure.

Recently a new, biologically safe technique called electromagnetic articulography has been introduced for the assessment of articulatory function. The electromagnetic articulograph uses alternating magnetic fields for tracking the movements of multiple points on supraglottic structures in the mid-sagittal plane and is capable of generating high resolution movement data required to study displacements, timing, speed and coordination of the articulators during speech. Although as yet electromagnetic articulography is purely a research tool, it has the potential to be used to monitor the effects of therapy aimed at improving articulatory function in speakers with MS. With further development, the procedure may also be able to provide real-time biofeedback to people with dysarthria associated with MS to aid in their relearning of tongue control during speech to enhance their overall intelligibility.

Physiological features of articulatory dysfunction in multiple sclerosis

Despite the frequent occurrence of articulatory dysfunction reported in American (Darley et al., 1972), Australian (FitzGerald et al., 1987) and Swedish (Hartelius et al., 1993) speakers with MS, few studies have investigated the nature of the physiological impairment in the articulatory mechanism of persons with MS. The most extensive study reported to date that utilized a range of specialized physiological instruments to assess the functioning of the lips and tongue in speakers with MS is that conducted by Murdoch et al. (1998). In that study, we used lip and tongue transduction systems to assess the physiological functioning of the articulators of 16 adults with MS. Since the publication of our original report in 1998, however, we have extended our study to include a further 17 subjects with MS. Consequently, the remainder of this section of the present chapter will focus on providing a synthesis of the findings of the expanded study, which until this time have not been published.

The subjects examined in our expanded study were 33 individuals with a diagnosis of definite MS. The diagnosis was made by a neurologist on the basis of a combination of neuroradiological and clinical signs. Of the 33 MS subjects, 10 were classified as being dysarthric by a speech/language pathologist and 23 were nondysarthric. None of the subjects included had a history of speech disturbance prior to diagnosis of MS. Likewise, none had any history of a co-existing neurological disorder or a speech disturbance due to a disorder occurring in addition to multiple sclerosis. Eighteen non-neurologically impaired individuals matched for age, sex and level of education served as controls. The personal and medical details of the 33 subjects with MS involved in the expanded study are presented in Table 4.1.

Table 4.1 Biographical and clinical details of the multiple sclerosis subjects

Subject number	Sex	Age# at assessment	Age# at diagnosis	Age# at onset	Duration# of MS	Type of MS	Signs and symptoms	Presence of dysarthria	Current medications
1	F	40	30	NDA	10	CP	Mobility problems, visual problems	No	Baclofen
2	F	42	29	16	26	RR	Sudden collapses, blindness during pregnancy, tremor cramping	No	Diabex, Diamicron, Becotide, Capoten
3	F	54	52	50	4	CP	Numbness, tingling, fine motor problems, weakness in legs, poor hearing, poor taste, blurred vision, short-term memory problems	No	Hormone Replacement Therapy
4	M	33	23	21	12	CP	Weakness (greater on left side), dysarthria	Yes	Methylprednisolone
5	M	62	57	57	5	CP	Optic neuritis, diplopia	No	Baclofen, Sinequan Hiprex, Rehipral,Baclofen, Prozac
6	F	35	19	17	18	CP	Poor mobility, visual deficits, incontinence, dysarthria	Yes	
7	F	49	34	34	15	NDA	Headaches, weakness in left leg, disorientation, paraesthesiae, bladder problems	No	Tryptanol, Renitec, Dyazide, Zantac
8	F	73	63	25	48	NDA	Bladder retention, paraesthesiae, pain, episodes of blindness, blurred vision, weak limbs	No	Enduron, Tegretol
9	F	45	45	45	<1	CP	Dysarthria, mobility problems	Yes	Prythyrodin
10	F	43	42	42	1.5	RR (remission)	Imbalance, fatigue	No	Diabex, Dinol, Naprosynj, Ditropan

11	M	39	38	35	4	RR (relapse)	Imbalance, fatigue, loss of control of left hand and left leg, dysarthria	Yes	None
12	F	50	27	26	24	CP	Dysarthria, right arm and leg numbness, left facial numbness, balance and movement problems	Yes	None
13	F	47	35	34	13	RR (relapse)	Blurred vision, swallowing, mobility problems	No	Baclofen, Steroids, Doxepin
14	M	49	45	40	9	CP	Pain in arms and legs, muscle cramping, poor vision, poor memory, balance problems, breathing problems	No	Dolvon, Prozac, Rivotril
15	F	43	43	43	<1	RR (remission)	Motor impairments, numbness in tongue sometimes	No	Prednisone, Steroids
16	F	45	38	28	17	RR (remission)	Numbness and weakness on right side, paraesthesiae on left side, unsteady gait, memory and word finding difficulties	No	None
17	M	44	31	NDA	13	NDA	General level of impairment is mild to moderate	NDA	NDA
18	F	54	34	NDA	20	RR, then CP	Difficulties with body temperature regulation, spasmodic asthma	NDA	None
19	F	57	35	15	42	RR	Loss of memory, poor coordination of thought and speech, blindness twice, swallowing problems, right side of tongue paralysis, (contd)	No	Prednisone

(contd)

Table 4.1 (contd)

Subject number	Sex	Age at assessment	Age at diagnosis	Age at onset	Duration of MS	Type of MS	Signs and symptoms	Presence of dysarthria	Current medications
							deaf in right ear, spasm of right side of chest, incontinent bowel, bladder retention, extreme fatigue, sharp muscular spasms		
20	F	56	54	34	22	NDA	Numbness left side of face and scalp/Neuralgia, loss of balance, double vision, nausea during attacks	No	Prothiden, Isoptin, Hormone replacement therapy, cholesterol treatment
21	M	55	48	48	7	CP	Depression, dysphagia (thickened fluids), hearing impairment (biaural aids), word finding difficulties.	No	Lovanf, Rivotril, Losec, Prepulsid, Coloxyl, Durolax, Alprazolam, Panamax
22	F	46	NDA	31	15	CP	Poor memory, fatigue, sensitive to heat, mobility problems, dysfluent, dysarthria	Yes	None
23	F	39	26	NDA	13	CP with relapse	Fatigue, cognitive ability, dizziness, balance problems, some mobility problems, speech slurred when tired	No	Betaferon
24	M	43	40	39	4	CP	Optic neuritis, pain, tremor and weakness in legs, poor breath control, speech problems when tired	No	Methotrexate
25	F	46	45	NDA	1	CP	Balance problems, dysarthria	Yes	None
26	F	58	NDA	35	23	NDA	Trigeminal neuralgia, dysphagia	No	NDA

27	F	41	34	28	13	RR	General weakness on right side, odd sensation in legs, difficulty with multisyllabic words, voice fades when tired	No	NDA
28	M	55	32	NDA	23	CP	Weakness in arms and legs, problems with eyes, mobility problems	No	NDA
29	F	51	44	NDA	7	RR	Slurred speech, balance problems, some trouble with legs	Yes	None
30	M	34	31	23	11	CP	Bilateral hearing loss wears aids, vision problems, foot drop, slurred speech, balance problems, short and long-term memory problems, wheelchair bound	Yes	Methotrexate, folic acid
31	F	43	26	NDA	17	RR	Lack of sensation, problems with eyes, twitch, mobility and balance problems, jumbled speech	No	Betaferon, Prednisolone
32	F	37	32	30	7	CP	Muscle weakness, balance problems, double vision left side, facial droop on left side, mobility problems	No	Betaferon
33	M	50	45	NDA	5	CP	Balance problems, speech problems, vision deteriorating, mobility problems, swallowing difficulties.	Yes	Methotrexate

Note: # = years; NDA = no data available; MS = multiple sclerosis; CP = chronically progressive; RR = relapsing/remitting

The physiological assessment of articulatory function involved measurement of tongue and lip strength, endurance and rate of repetitive movements using pressure transduction systems. The transducer for assessing tongue function was identical to the rubber-bulb pressure transducer described by Murdoch, Attard and Ozanne (1995). The transducer enabled estimation of tongue strength, endurance and fine motor control during performance of a range of different non-speech tasks.

A miniaturized pressure transducer based on semi-conductor strain-gauge technology similar to that described by Hinton and Luschei (1992) was used to estimate each subject's lip strength and endurance. For a detailed description of the lip pressure transducer and the procedure for its use the reader is referred to Thompson et al. (1997). The transducer allowed direct measurement of the contact pressure between the lips during performance of six different non-speech tasks yielding estimates of lip strength, endurance and fine motor control.

The results of the physiological assessment of tongue function showed that, as a group, the subjects with MS presented with significantly impaired tongue function based on strength, endurance and rate measures, compared to the control group. Specifically, the MS group performed significantly below the control subjects on all measures of tongue function with the exception of the three measures relating to fine motor control. On none of the tasks, however, were the dysarthric MS subjects found to differ significantly from the non-dysarthric MS subjects.

Reduced muscle strength is a frequently documented symptom of MS. The nature of muscle weakness in MS was investigated by Rice et al. (1992). They used electromyography to examine the quadriceps muscles of a group of MS patients and found that the muscle forces are weak and that the muscles could not be activated maximally. Rice et al. (1992) also found that the demyelination associated with MS led to reduced maximum motoneurone firing rates which could conceivably account for the reduction of muscle strength (Rice et al., 1992). During maximal contraction of the quadriceps muscle, Rice et al. (1992) observed that firing rates rarely exceeded 17 Hz in MS subjects compared to 24 Hz for normals. It is possible that, in a similar way, reduced motoneurone firing rates could account, at least in part, for the diminished tongue strength exhibited by the MS subjects examined in our study.

Muscle weakness in persons with MS has also been attributed to increased central motor conduction times (Hess et al., 1987). Central motor conduction time is measured by obtaining the latency differences in responses from a particular muscle to magnetic stimulation of the motor cortex. Hess et al. (1987) studied central motor conduction times in MS patients with weakness of the abductor muscle of the little finger, and found that muscle weakness was highly correlated with an increased central motor conduction time. Other researchers have also documented increased central motor conduction time in subjects with MS (Mills and Murray, 1985; Hess et al., 1986). It is therefore conceivable that increased central motor conduction times could also be a contributing factor to the decreased lingual strength identified in the MS group in the current study.

The MS subjects investigated in our study demonstrated reduced tongue and lip endurance compared to the control subjects based on their performance on the sustained submaximal tongue and lip pressure tasks. These results are suggestive of fatigue of the lingual and lip muscles during performance of this task. Several researchers have discussed mechanisms of muscle fatigue in MS which may to some degree account for the reduced endurance of tongue and lip strength observed in our group of MS subjects (Lehman et al., 1989; Sharma et al., 1995). Central sources of fatigue are considered to be a contributing factor for MS patients, and could involve at least two different mechanisms. First, as noted above, firing rates of motor neurones can be decreased because of lesions in corticospinal pathways, resulting in muscle fatigue (Rice et al., 1992; Kent-Braun et al., 1994a). Secondly, reaction times are delayed and cognitive activity is abnormal in many patients with MS, suggesting that the processes involved in preparing for and initiating motor responses may also be affected (Sandroni et al., 1992; Sharma et al., 1995).

Recent studies have also shown that peripheral fatigue is evident in MS subjects (Kent-Braun et al., 1994b; Sharma et al., 1995). Kent-Braun et al. (1994b) found that MS patients exhibited reduced muscular oxidative capacity, as evidenced by slowed phosphocreatine resynthesis following exercise (phosphocreatine is a store of high-energy phosphate in muscles and therefore is an energy source for muscular contraction). It is therefore possible that both central and peripheral factors may have contributed to the observed reductions in tongue and lip endurance of the MS subjects in the present study.

The performance of the MS subjects on the fast tongue and lip pressure repetition tasks revealed that the MS subjects produced significantly fewer repetitions during the 10-second time period, indicating an impaired rate of tongue and lip movement. The reduction in rate of repetitive tongue movements is probably a direct result of the impairments in tongue strength and endurance noted above. Luschei (1991) stated that reductions in strength may be particularly related to the speed of tongue movement during speech. He reported that, as tongue strength is decreased, the maximal attainable shortening velocity of the muscle fibres is decreased, and thus a reduction in the rate of movement results (Luschei, 1991). It is, therefore, possible that the lingual weakness identified in the present MS subjects may have led to their decreased rate of tongue movements. As will be evident from the discussion below, the same explanation could not be applied to the decrease in repetitive movement of the lips.

In contrast to the finding in relation to the tongue, lip strength was not significantly reduced in the MS group suggesting that MS affects the motor pathways to the tongue to a greater extent than the motor pathways to the lip muscles. The pattern of differential impairment of the tongue and lips observed in relation to maintenance of strength is consistent with studies of other neurological conditions. Several instrumental studies have investigated lip and tongue function in amyotrophic lateral sclerosis (Carpenter et al., 1978; De Paul et al., 1988; De Paul and Brooks, 1993; Langmore and Lehman, 1994) and reported that the tongue is significantly more impaired than the lips and jaw. Greater impairment of tongue function, compared to the lips and jaw, has also been documented in Parkinson's disease (Barlow and Abbs, 1983; Abbs et al., 1987). Barlow and Abbs (1983) suggested that there is a substantial physiological/neurophysiological basis for differential impairment of the articulatory subsystem as the labial, lingual and mandibular subsystems exhibit different biomechanical properties. The finding of differential impairment in relation to tongue and lip strength in our cohort of MS subjects further highlights the importance of assessing each component of the speech production apparatus independently to more accurately define the nature of the underlying pathophysiological deficits of the articulation disorder.

The physiological assessments also demonstrated pre-clinical signs of lingual and lip dysfunction in the non-dysarthric MS subjects. Specifically, although the non-dysarthric MS subjects exhibited perceptually normal speech, they recorded significantly reduced rates of repetitive tongue movements and decreased endurance compared to controls. Likewise they also exhibited significantly reduced lip endurance in comparison to the control subjects. Based on our findings it would appear that physiological assessments have the potential to detect deterioration in articulatory function caused by demyelination of nerve connections to the tongue and lip muscles, prior to any symptoms being perceived in the speech of persons with MS. This finding is consistent with that of Hartelius et al. (1993) who found that their non-dysarthric MS subjects had significantly impaired oromotor performance (on lips, jaw and tongue tasks) in the presence of perceptually normal articulation.

In conclusion, the physiological assessments confirmed that patients with MS demonstrate impaired articulatory abilities. In particular, the findings of our expanded study suggest that although both tongue and lip function are compromised, the impairment in tongue function is more severe and more encompassing than the disorder in lip function. Consequently, it is suggested that tongue dysfunction may be the primary cause of the perceived articulatory abnormalities in persons with MS and therefore should be a primary target for therapy. The presence of pre-clinical signs of articulatory dysfunction in the non-dysarthric MS cases, as identified by both the physiological and perceptual tests, highlights the need for careful monitoring of articulatory function in non-dysarthric MS persons and the possibility of the need to initiate therapy early in the course of the disease (see Chapter 6).

Velopharyngeal dysfunction in multiple sclerosis

During the process of speech production the velopharyngeal mechanism operates to modify the ratio of acoustic coupling between the oral and nasal cavities (Zemlin, 1988). In English speakers, velopharyngeal closure is achieved during the production of oral sounds, with the exclusion of the nasal consonants /m/, /n/ and /ng/, and vowels in close proximity to these consonants (Enderby et al., 1984). When the port is open (e.g. during nasal consonant production), air and vocal vibrations are permitted to expand into the nasal cavity effecting an increase in nasal resonance. Closure of the velopharyngeal port also influences articulatory proficiency by facilitating an increase in intra-oral pressure. Consequently, during speech production velopharyngeal insufficiency can manifest as hypernasality and/or articulatory imprecision.

Perceptual features of velopharyngeal dysfunction in multiple sclerosis

Hypernasality has been reported to be the most characteristic symptom of inadequate velopharyngeal closure (Isshiki et al., 1968) brought about by the inappropriate diversion of acoustic energy into the nasal cavity, resulting in excessively nasal speech (McWilliams et al., 1990). Although not a consistent perceptual feature of the dysarthria exhibited by individuals with MS, hypernasality has been reported to occur in the speech of a number of individuals with MS. Darley et al. (1972) documented the presence of perceptually hypernasal speech in 41 of their 168 (24%) MS subjects. Based on a perceptual analysis of a speech sample, FitzGerald et al. (1987) identified hypernasal resonance in 16 of their 23 (70%) MS subjects. In the expanded study of 56 persons with MS recently completed by the authors of the present chapter, 41% were identified as exhibiting hypernasal speech.

More recently, Hartelius et al. (1993) reported the presence of perceptually hypernasal speech in 8 out of their 30 (27%) MS subjects.

Other authors, however, have represented hypernasality as a rather insignificant item on long check-lists of speech features commonly associated with MS (Farmakides and Boone, 1960; Hartelius and Svensson, 1994). Given that hypernasality is often misperceived in traditionally applied, perceptual assessments of dysarthria due to the difficulty in perceptually isolating this deviant speech dimension from other speech features (Moll, 1970; Brancewicz and Reich, 1989) confirmation of velopharyngeal insufficiency in MS using physiological procedures is required.

Physiological assessment of velopharyngeal function in multiple sclerosis

A wide range of instrumental techniques are available to assess the functioning of the velopharyngeal valve in speakers with MS. Basically the different instruments available for this purpose can be divided into those that involve direct assessment and those that involve indirect assessment of the functioning of the velum. Direct assessment of the velopharyngeal mechanism predominantly involves radiographic and endoscopic techniques. Radiographic procedures, specifically cineradiographic and videofluoroscopic methods, display the dynamics of velopharyngeal closure on motion film (cineradiography) or videotape (videofluroscopy) which demonstrate the coordinated interaction of the velum and pharyngeal walls. Abnormalities of structure and function may be detected using these visually direct methods of investigation. The use of radiographic procedures, however, is limited somewhat by the laborious analysis procedures involved and by the need to expose patients to radiation.

Functioning of the velopharyngeal valve can also be observed directly by way of endoscopic procedures. A view of the velopharyngeal mechanism is most commonly achieved via transnasal insertion (nasoendoscopy) of a flexible endoscope into the nasopharynx via the nasal passages, allowing the velopharyngeal region to be viewed from above. The nasoendoscopic procedure does not impair normal articulatory movements and therefore allows for the direct observation of velar movement during speech. This type of direct investigation can provide important information regarding deficits in timing and in coordination of velopharyngeal closure as well as identify sluggish, reduced or incomplete palatal movement. The nasoendoscope can be used in conjunction with a video recording system (videonasoendoscopy) to enable the image to be saved for later analysis.

Indirect methods for assessing the functioning of the velopharyngeal valve include nasal airflow and air pressure techniques, photodetection methods, nasal/oral acoustic emissions and nasal accelerometry.

Measures of nasal airflow can be achieved through the use of a pneumo-tachograph or a warm-wire anemometer (Hutters and Brondsted, 1992). These devices can be either fitted to a nasal mask or connected to a plastic catheter placed in one nostril. Unfortunately, the nasal airflows cannot be used as an index of the degree of nasalization during speech, as nasal airflow reflects many aspects of vocal tract function such as changing intraoral pressures, oral port constrictions and nasal resistance (Baken, 1987). Despite this limitation, nasal airflow can be useful in the gross differentiation of good, fair and poor velopharyngeal function.

Photodetection methods involve the introduction of light into the oral cavity and its subsequent transmission and detection in the region above the velopharyngeal port (McWilliams et al., 1990). The amount of light detected during a specific speech task is proportional to the size of the velopharyngeal orifice (Moon and Lagu, 1987).

Another indirect method of assessing velopharyngeal function is based on determination of the ratio of acoustic output from the oral and nasal cavities. This system is commercially marketed as the 'Nasometer'. The acoustic signal input is achieved through two directional micro-phones, one situated at the level of the nasal cavity and the other in front of the oral cavity. These two microphones are separated by an efficient sound separator plate. As the speech signal is entered into the system, the ratio of nasal to oral plus nasal acoustic energy is calculated in terms of percentage as a 'nasalance' score. Subtle changes in the degree of nasality are reflected in the nasalance percentage. The Nasometer is a further development and adaptation of TONAR (The Oral Nasal Acoustic Ratio) technique developed by Fletcher (1970).

Nasal accelerometry is based on the principle that, as nasal sounds cause vibrations of the soft tissue of the nose, then an accelerometer (a transducer sensitive to vibration) placed on the nose could be used to detect nasalization. The technique most commonly employed involves the placement of miniature accelerometers upon the lateral nasal carti-lage and thyroid lamina, which detect nasal and laryngeal vibrations produced during speech. The magnitudes of the vibrations detected are then used to calculate a ratio of nasal to laryngeal vibration, providing an index of nasality, the Horii Oral Nasal Coupling (HONC) index (Horii, 1983).

Physiological features of velopharyngeal dysfunction in multiple sclerosis

Due to the quantifiable data provided by instrumental assessments combined with the reported unreliability and poor validity of perceptual judgements of nasality (Van Demark et al., 1985), the contemporary approach to the diagnosis of velopharyngeal inadequacy encompasses the amalgamation of both subjective (perceptual based) and objective (instrument based) techniques. Unfortunately, to date only one study has been reported that has utilized physiological instruments to assess velopharyngeal function in speakers with MS (Darley et al., 1972). To address this lack of objective studies the authors of the present chapter have recently completed a physiological analysis of velopharyngeal function in a group of 33 individuals with MS using nasal accelerometry. The remainder of the present chapter is devoted to providing a synthesis of the findings of this analysis.

The subjects examined were the same 33 cases with MS described previously in this chapter (see Table 4.1). Thirty-three non-neurologically impaired individuals matched for age, sex and level of education served as controls. Physiological evaluation of velopharyngeal function was conducted using a nasal accelerometry technique. The nasal accelerometry technique involved the use of two miniature accelerometers one placed on the lateral nasal cartilage and the other over the larynx, designed to detect nasal and throat vibrations during speech. The output signals from the respective accelerometers were relayed to a computerized physiological data acquisition system and the magnitudes of the vibrations used to calculate a ratio of nasal to laryngeal vibrations, thereby providing an index of nasality referred to as the Horii Oral Nasal Coupling (HONC) index (Horii, 1983). For each subject the vibratory measurements were recorded during production of a series of nasal and non-nasal sounds, words and sentences. For a complete description of the nasal accelerometry procedure the reader is referred to Theodoros et al. (1993).

The results of the nasal accelerometry assessment revealed that, as a group, the MS subjects failed to demonstrate significantly different levels of nasality compared to the matched controls across the various speech tasks thereby indicating that their nasal resonance was within normal limits. In addition, comparison of the HONC indices achieved by the 10 dysarthric MS subjects with those of the non-dysarthric MS subjects also showed no significant differences in nasality between these two subject groups. Consequently, the dysarthric MS subjects examined in our study were no more nasal than the non-dysarthric MS or control subjects suggesting that, although impaired in other subsystems of the speech production mechanism, their velopharyngeal function was intact.

Although the group data failed to detect the presence of velopharyngeal dysfunction in either the dysarthric or non-dysarthric MS groups, examination of the nasal accelerometry data on an individual subject basis revealed that one MS subject (subject 16) consistently demonstrated elevated nasality levels across the various non-nasal speech tasks (non-nasal sounds, words, sentences and utterances) when compared to the relevant control group mean. The small proportion of instrumentally detected hypernasal subjects identified in our study is generally consistent with the results of the only other documented objective evaluation of velopharyngeal function in MS. Using oral manometry, Darley et al. (1972) confirmed the presence of velopharyngeal dysfunction in only 3 of their 155 (2%) MS subjects.

The findings of our physiological analysis of velopharyngeal function in MS reported here cast some doubt on the validity of reports in the literature of a moderate (27%) (Hartelius et al., 1993) to high (70%) (FitzGerald et al., 1987) incidence of velopharyngeal inadequacy in MS speakers based on perceptual analyses. Rather our findings support the observations of Van Demark et al. (1985) who reported that the vocal feature of nasality may in fact be perceived in the presence or absence of velopharyngeal inadequacy, rendering this perceptual feature an unreliable index of velopharyngeal function. As noted by other authors, the vocal feature of hypernasality may be influenced by numerous secondary speech characteristics during perceptual evaluation of speech, such as articulatory proficiency, pitch, loudness, pleasantness and linguistic skill (Moll, 1970; Brancewicz and Reich, 1989). Clinically our findings suggest that, prior to speech pathologists initiating therapy aimed at remediating a perceived velopharyngeal inadequacy in MS speakers, they take steps to confirm their perceptual findings by way of an objective, instrumental analysis of velopharyngeal function. Only after such confirmation should they proceed to implement therapy aimed at reducing perceived levels of hypernasality.

In conclusion, although velopharyngeal dysfunction may occur in individuals with MS, it would appear that its incidence is low, occurring in only a small percentage of the MS population. Given, however, that the data presented above were collected from cases with predominantly either mild or moderate MS it is possible that a higher incidence of velopharyngeal insufficiency might occur in individuals with more severe MS symptoms. Certainly further research using a larger cohort of MS cases, including more individuals with a more severe form of the disease, is warranted to determine the relationship between disease severity and the manifestation of velopharyngeal dysfunction. Also of interest were the findings in relation to subject 16. Although she failed to exhibit a perceptible dysarthria (see Table 4.1) subject 16 did demonstrate velopharyngeal inadequacy as determined by the nasal accelerometry technique. While this finding lends very limited support to the hypothesis of preclinical velopharyngeal dysfunction in persons with MS, it highlights the need for future research involving follow-up, longitudinal investigations to monitor changes in the status of velopharyngeal function concurrent with disease progression.

Chapter 5
Laryngeal and respiratory dysfunction in multiple sclerosis

DEBORAH G THEODOROS, BRUCE E MURDOCH AND
ELIZABETH C WARD

Introduction

The laryngeal and respiratory subsystems of the speech mechanism produce the basic energy source for speech production. In that these subsystems are interdependent in the process of speech production, dysfunction in either or both of these two subsystems may result in insufficient breath support for speech and/or inefficient phonatory function. The subsequent impairment in speech production may be manifested in a variety of forms, including shortened phrase length due to a reduction in expiratory air flow, impaired control of pitch and loudness, abnormal vocal quality, and impairments in the general stress patterning in speech.

Although there have been a number of studies which have investigated the laryngeal and respiratory function in a variety of neurologically disordered individuals, sparse attention has been paid to defining the perceptual and physiological features of these particular subsystems of the speech production mechanism in persons with MS. A review of previous and recent research relating to the laryngeal and respiratory subsystems in persons with MS will be provided in the following sections.

Laryngeal dysfunction in multiple sclerosis

Phonatory dysfunction has been identified as one of the most prevalent impairments in speech production demonstrated by various MS populations around the world (see Chapter 2). As early as 1916, Scripture suggested the presence of abnormal laryngeal function in MS subjects based on phonoautographic evidence of irregularities in the tension of the vocal cords during vocalization. Since this time, a number of authors have reported on a wide range and level of severity of phonatory disorders in persons with MS. To date, the assessment of laryngeal function in MS populations has mainly focused on perceptual (see Chapter 2) and acoustic evaluation (see Chapter 3) with minimal attention being given to analyses of the physiological bases of the phonatory disturbances.

Perceptual features of laryngeal dysfunction in multiple sclerosis

In a review of 82 MS subjects, Farmakides and Boone (1960) identified impaired pitch variation and poor phonatory control (initiation and cessation of voicing) as contributing factors to the subjects' dysarthria. It was suggested that these abnormal phonatory features were due to impaired control of fine movements of the larynx. The most comprehensive investigation of the speech production in persons with MS, however, was conducted by Darley et al. (1972) who found that harshness was the second most frequently occurring deviant speech feature (72%) in a sample of 168 individuals, 41% of whom were dysarthric. In addition, other abnormal phonatory disturbances including impaired pitch control (37%) and inappropriate pitch level (24%) were also apparent in the speech output of these individuals. A comparable occurrence of dysphonia (73%) in the form of a 'creaky voice' was identified by Hartelius et al. (1993) in their group of 30 Swedish subjects with MS (47% dysarthric). One third of the subjects in this study exhibited an inappropriate pitch level with a further one-third being perceived to demonstrate a breathy vocal quality. In a larger cohort of 77 subjects with MS, glottal fry and harshness were found to be two of the most predominant deviant speech features evident in this population, with glottal fry occurring in 88% of the subjects and harshness in 86% of the group. Glottal fry was noted to be present to a mild degree in the majority of these individuals exhibiting this speech feature. Eighty per cent of the subjects exhibited a mildly harsh vocal quality, while 20% of the subjects demonstrated a moderately harsh vocal quality. A strained-strangled vocal quality and hoarseness were also perceived to be present in 62% and 16% of the subjects, respectively (Hartelius et al., 1999, 2000).

In another study by Hartelius, Buder and Strand (1997), in which 30% of the 20 subjects with MS were dysarthric, a number of different forms of phonatory disturbances were identified. Approximately 35% of the subjects were rated as exhibiting a hoarse-harsh vocal quality in comparison to 30% of the subjects who demonstrated a predominantly harsh voice. Twenty-five per cent of the subjects were considered to have a breathy component to their voices (breathy, breathy-normal, breathy-hoarse), while a further two (10%) subjects were perceived to exhibit either a harsh-strained strangled or a normal-hoarse vocal quality.

For Australian speakers with MS, harshness has been identified as the most predominant phonatory disturbance in a group of 56 subjects examined by the authors, occurring in almost half of the group (47%). Hoarseness and reduced pitch steadiness were perceived to be present in 39% of the subjects with other parameters of vocal quality such as breathiness, glottal fry, and strained-strangled voice evident in 38%, 36%, and 30%, respectively. Prosodic features associated with laryngeal dysfunction, including reduced variation of pitch and inappropriate pitch level were noted to be evident in approximately 50% of the subjects with MS while impaired variation and level of loudness were identified in 38% and 27 % of the subjects, respectively. Similarly, on the Frenchay Dysarthria Assessment (Enderby, 1983), a subgroup of 30 MS subjects demonstrated a mild impairment of the laryngeal subsystem in relation to vocal quality, phonation time, and pitch and loudness variability. The MS subjects were found to be significantly more impaired on each of the subsystem parameters, compared to the control group.

The range of phonatory features reported in the literature reflects the diversity of the phonatory disorders perceived to be present in the MS population. The exact nature of these phonatory disturbances, however, will not be determined until full physiological investigation of the laryngeal mechanism is undertaken to ascertain the bases of the various vocal features.

Physiological assessment of laryngeal function in multiple sclerosis

A number of physiological methods of assessment of laryngeal function in persons with MS are currently available both clinically and in research laboratories. These assessment techniques involve the use of a range of instrumentation designed to perform either direct or indirect examination of laryngeal function in relation to vocal fold movement, laryngeal musculature, vocal fold vibratory patterns, and laryngeal aerodynamics.

Clinically, the most widely used instrumental technique for the assessment of vocal fold movement is direct laryngoscopy which utilizes either a rigid endoscope positioned posteriorly in the oral cavity or a flexible fibrescope passed through the nose and situated in the oropharynx and hypopharynx. Both the rigid endoscope and the flexible fibrescope are connected to a video recording system which allows the examiner to monitor the position of the instruments and the movement of the vocal folds. The flexible fibrescope laryngoscopy offers the most comprehensive examination of laryngeal function in that the oral cavity is not obstructed during this procedure and vocal fold movements during a range of normal speech tasks and singing can be readily observed (Baken, 1987; Colton and Casper, 1996). To achieve a more detailed examination of vocal fold movement and vibratory behaviour, a stroboscopic light source is often used in direct laryngoscopy. The stroboscopic light emits rapid pulses which, when equal to the vocal frequency, will result in the vocal folds appearing to be at a standstill. Alternatively, if the frequency of the pulses is greater or less than the vocal frequency, the vocal folds will appear to move in slow motion allowing the examiner to observe finer details of vocal fold vibration and movement. Videostroboscopy provides considerable information in relation to symmetry of vocal fold vibration, glottal closure, regularity of successive vibrations, horizontal excursion of the vocal folds, status of the mucosal wave, phase closure, and the presence of any non-vibratory sections of the vocal folds (Colton and Casper, 1996). The use of videostroboscopy in the assessment of laryngeal function in MS has not been fully explored. However, the potential of this technique to provide a detailed and accurate assessment of vocal fold vibration and movement, and to document changes associated with the progression of the disease, is considerable.

Another direct physiological assessment of laryngeal function which may be useful for the MS population is electromyography (EMG) which measures the electrical activity of the laryngeal musculature. The technique involves the use of either surface or indwelling electrodes to record electrical potentials generated by the laryngeal muscles. Surface electrodes placed on the larynx provide information concerning the global activity of the laryngeal muscles rather than information regarding specific muscles as achieved when using indwelling electrodes. As such, EMG using surface electrodes may provide information concerning the degree of tension in the laryngeal musculature in persons with MS. The use of indwelling electrodes situated in specific muscles of the larynx, however, will provide a more detailed assessment of laryngeal muscle function in individuals with MS as specific electromyographic manifestations of muscle activity have been identified in neurologically disordered patients. These features include increased or decreased amplitudes of muscle activity, extraneous bursts of muscle activity, and reduced or increased muscle activation (Colton and Casper, 1996).

One of the most popular indirect methods of assessing the vibratory pattern of the vocal folds is electroglottography (EGG), which is non-invasive and readily performed on persons with varying degrees of neurological disorder, including persons with MS. Electroglottography measures vocal fold contact area based on the capacity of human tissue to conduct an electric current. A low current signal is passed between two electrodes positioned on the thyroid lamina. The flow of the current between the two electrodes varies when the vocal folds are adducted and abducted to varying degrees. The varying electrical impedance is displayed in the form of a glottal waveform depicting the opening and closing phases of the vibratory cycle of the vocal folds (Gilbert et al., 1984; Baken, 1987). Both qualitative and quantitative analyses of the waveform have been reported extensively in the literature (Colton and Conture, 1990; Colton and Casper, 1996). Measures taken from the glottal waveform have included fundamental frequency, duty cycle (ratio of open phase to total glottal cycle), closing time (period of time from the lowest point in the open phase to the highest point in the closed phase), and slope of closure. Although this technique may yield useful information concerning vocal fold vibratory patterns, there are a sufficient number of factors which limit the effectiveness of this assessment (head movements, neck tissue thickness, electrode placement, skin-electrode resistance, and changes in laryngeal height during speech) to cause many researchers in the field to advocate for caution in the interpretation of EGG results (Gilbert et al., 1984; Hanson et al., 1988; Colton and Conture, 1990). Different types of EGG instrumentation including the Voicescope, the Laryngograph, the F-J Electroglottograph, and the Synchrovoice Quantitative Electroglottograph (Baken, 1987) are available to obtain EGG measures of vocal fold vibration.

A similar measure of glottal area may be obtained using a different technique known as photoglottography in which light is directed from above the larynx and through the glottis where it is detected by a light-sensitive device positioned over the outer surface of the trachea, below the vocal folds (Colton and Casper, 1996). The amount of light detected by the device varies according to the degree of opening and closing of the glottis, revealing an approximation of glottal area (Baken, 1987). Parameters measured during this procedure include the speed quotient (speed of opening phase divided by the speed of the closing phase) and open quotient (time of the open phase divided by the total period of vibration). Although photoglottography has application in the assessment of vibratory patterns in persons with MS, EGG is clinically more readily available for use as an assessment device.

The laryngeal aerodynamics of persons with MS involves the assessment of parameters such as phonatory flow, subglottal pressure, and laryngeal resistance to air flow during speech. A variety of techniques have been developed to measure each of these parameters of vocal tract aerodynamics. Although measurement of laryngeal aerodynamics provides useful diagnostic and therapeutic information, intra-subject variability is inherent within this aspect of assessment of laryngeal function, necessitating several recordings for each subject to obtain reliable physiological measurement (Hammen and Yorkston, 1994). Phonatory flow may be measured using a range of instrumentation, including pneumotachographs, hot-wire anemometers, plethysmographs, electroaerometers, and differential oropharyngeal pressure catheters (Miller and Daniloff, 1993), while subglottal pressure is assessed indirectly using a polyethylene tube inserted into the oral cavity and connected to a differential pressure transducer (Netsell and Hixon, 1978). Laryngeal subglottal pressure is considered equal to the intra-oral pressure produced during the production of a voiceless stop consonant. Laryngeal airway resistance is a mathematical derivative determined by calculating the ratio of subglottal pressure to phonatory air flow rate and requires the simultaneous recording of these two parameters of laryngeal aerodynamics (Smitheran and Hixon, 1981; Hoit and Hixon, 1992). A commercially available voice function analyser, the Aerophone II (Kay Elemetrics), can now provide measurement of most aspects of laryngeal aerodynamics within the clinical situation. This instrument consists of a hand-held face mask and transducer module incorporating transducers for recording airflow, intra-oral pressure, and sound pressure level. The associated software program produces additional measurements of laryngeal airway resistance, glottal efficiency and a range of other parameters (Frokjaer-Jensen, 1992). As the Aerophone II has been utilized in studies involving neurologically disordered subjects and found to provide useful research and clinical information (Murdoch et al.,1994; Theodoros and Murdoch, 1994), it has potential for use in the assessment of laryngeal function in persons with MS.

The objective information obtained from physiological methods of assessment of laryngeal function provides a more detailed level of analysis not achieved through perceptual evaluation. In particular, instrumental assessment techniques are more effective in determining the underlying laryngeal pathophysiology in neurologically impaired persons in which progressive damage to various levels of the nervous system results in a complex array of subjective perceptual features.

Physiological features of laryngeal dysfunction in multiple sclerosis

Apart from Scripture's (1916) early investigation of vocal fold tension in subjects with MS, there have not been any reports of physiological investigations of laryngeal function in persons with MS. The lack of physiological assessment of laryngeal function in MS may be due to a number of factors, including availability of instrumentation and the progressive nature of the disease. The need for such evaluation, however, is imperative if treatment programmes are to be designed to accurately target the underlying physiological impairment within the laryngeal subsystem.

In an attempt to overcome the dearth of information regarding the physiological nature of laryngeal dysfunction in MS, a group of 33 persons with MS was recently assessed by the authors to determine the status of laryngeal function in this population. Biographical and clinical details relating to these subjects were presented in the previous chapter (see Table 4.1). Ten of these subjects demonstrated a dysarthric speech disturbance ranging in severity from mild to severe while the remaining 23 individuals with MS did not exhibit any perceptible dysarthria. Physiological methods of assessment included electroglottography (Fourcin Laryngograph) and an assessment of laryngeal aerodynamics (Aerophone II voice function analyser). Electroglottographic measures included fundamental frequency, duty cycle, and closing time, while measures of laryngeal aerodynamics consisted of subglottal pressure, phonatory air flow, sound pressure level, glottal resistance, and ad/abduction rate of the vocal folds. The results of these assessments revealed that the MS group as a whole were not significantly different to the control group on any of the electroglottographic or aerodynamic parameters. In addition, there were no significant differences detected on these parameters between the subgroups of MS dysarthric speakers, the MS non-dysarthric speakers, and the control subjects. The lack of statistically significant differences amongst the three groups most likely reflected the small number of MS dysarthric speakers, the mild degree of impairment evident in the majority of these subjects, and the intersubject variability evident in the EGG and laryngeal aerodynamic data.

Although the group data failed to identify laryngeal dysfunction in the MS subjects, examination of the data on an individual basis revealed that several of the MS dysarthric speakers did, in fact, demonstrate impairments in laryngeal function compared to the control group. Six (60%) dysarthric speakers exhibited some abnormality of the vibratory pattern of the vocal folds during the production of vowel and/or consonant prolongations that were at least one standard deviation above or below the control group mean across a minimum of two parameters. The patterns of impairment identified from the EGG assessment were consistent with both hyper- and hypofunctioning laryngeal behaviours, distributed equally amongst the six dysarthric speakers. Similarly, examination of the aerodynamic data for each of the 10 dysarthric speakers revealed that six (60%) of these subjects demonstrated impairments in laryngeal aerodynamics which were at least one standard deviation above or below control values for any one of the parameters measured. Reduced subglottal pressure was identified as the predominant aerodynamic deficit, occurring in four of the subjects. Phonatory airflow was found to be reduced in two persons and increased in another individual while decreases in glottal resistance and sound pressure level occurred in single subjects. As has been the case in other neurologically disordered populations, it would appear that the evaluation of laryngeal function in persons with MS may require examination of the individual data to identify impairment in vibratory patterns and laryngeal aerodynamics.

Subclinical manifestations of laryngeal dysfunction in multiple sclerosis

As previously mentioned in Chapter 2, subclinical manifestations of laryngeal dysfunction as determined perceptually have been identified in persons with MS who do not exhibit a dysarthric speech disturbance (Hartelius et al., 1993). Similarly, the non-dysarthric MS subjects investigated in our study, using the FDA, were found to be significantly impaired in relation to phonation time, pitch and loudness variability, and vocal quality, compared to the control subjects.

Although these subclinical perceptual manifestations of laryngeal dysfunction were not confirmed physiologically in the non-dysarthric MS subjects as a group, closer examination of the data on an individual basis revealed that a number of the subjects demonstrated abnormal vocal fold vibratory patterns and laryngeal aerodynamics, compared to the control group. Of the 23 non-dysarthric MS subjects investigated in the authors' study, nine (39%) subjects demonstrated abnormal vocal fold vibratory patterns involving at least two EGG parameters while 16 (69%) subjects exhibited abnormal laryngeal aerodynamics on at least one parameter. The variability evident in the EGG and laryngeal aerodynamic data recorded for the non-dysarthric MS subjects was consistent with the failure to achieve statistically significant differences between this group and the control subjects. The results, however, suggest that some persons with MS begin to demonstrate physiological deficits in the laryngeal subsystem prior to the perceptual manifestation of a dysarthric speech disturbance. This finding is consistent with that of Yorkston, Miller and Strand (1995) who reported that changes in vocal quality were typical of the mild dysarthria initially presenting in persons with MS. Further research involving larger groups of non-dysarthric MS subjects, however, is required to comprehensively evaluate the presence and nature of physiological subclinical features of laryngeal dysfunction in this group of MS individuals.

Respiratory dysfunction in multiple sclerosis

One of the earliest observations of respiratory dysfunction in persons with MS was reported by Farmakides and Boone (1960) who noted that the weak voices of patients with MS appeared to be due to a general disturbance in respiration involving poor control of exhalation. To date, the limited number of studies in the speech pathology literature which have investigated respiratory function in MS have largely been subjective, perceptual accounts of this aspect of the speech mechanism.

Perceptual features of respiratory dysfunction in multiple sclerosis

In their study of the speech of 168 MS patients, Darley et al. (1972) indirectly identified respiratory dysfunction in this population as being associated with impaired loudness control (77%), increased breathiness in speech (22%), and decreases in the duration of vowel prolongations. Both impaired loudness control and increased breathiness were accompanied by decreases in vital capacity (35%) in the MS subjects. In the Swedish study of 77 MS subjects by Hartelius et al. (1999, 2000), approximately three-quarters (77%) of the subjects were perceived to exhibit impaired respiratory support for speech with 74% of these subjects demonstrating a mild impairment and 26% of the cohort exhibiting a moderate to severe reduction in this deviant speech dimension. Impairment in respiratory function in Swedish subjects with MS has also been identified using a clinical dysarthria assessment tool developed by Hartelius et al. (1993), which uses both speech and nonspeech tasks. In this study, both the MS subjects as a total group and the 14 dysarthric speakers were found to be significantly impaired in respiratory function compared to normal controls. On maximum performance tasks involving expiratory pressure and sustained breath control, the MS subjects were not found to be significantly different to the controls, although the values recorded for the individuals with MS were lower than those recorded for their control counterparts (Hartelius et al., 1993).

In a study of a group of 56 Australian speakers with MS recently completed in the authors' own laboratory, impaired breath support for speech was identified perceptually in 52% of the subjects. The majority (66%) of these individuals exhibited a mild impairment of breath support, while the remaining 34% of the subjects were perceived to demonstrate moderate to severe reductions in breath support. In support of these perceptual findings, the results of a Frenchay Dysarthria Assessment (FDA) (Enderby, 1983) of the respiratory subsystem in a subgroup of 30 of these MS subjects (all subjects in Table 4.1 except for Subjects 3, 14, 19) revealed the presence of a mild, yet significant, impairment of respiratory function in persons with MS compared to control subjects. Ten of the individuals with MS in this study exhibited a dysarthric speech disturbance (see Table 4.1). These latter individuals also demonstrated a significant impairment in respiratory function of similar severity, at rest and during speech, compared to the control subjects.

The results of the perceptual assessments of respiratory function in persons with MS to date have indicated that, in general, more than half of a population of persons with MS will demonstrate features of respiratory dysfunction to a predominantly mild degree. Physiologically based instrumental assessment of respiration, however, is required to confirm these perceptual findings and to define the specific physiological impairments (e.g. inadequate breath supply, poor expiratory control) underlying the respiratory dysfunction evident in persons with MS.

Physiological assessment of respiratory function in multiple sclerosis

Although there has been limited research into the physiological basis of respiratory dysfunction in persons with MS, a range of objective instrumental methods are available to facilitate such analyses. The main aspects of respiratory function assessed instrumentally involve direct measurements of lung capacity and indirect measurements of the movements of the chest wall during speech production.

Measures of respiratory volumes may be readily obtained using clinical spirometric techniques which are non-invasive and simple to administer. During maximum effort tasks, air is blown into a tube or face mask attached to a spirometer which records a range of parameters, including vital capacity (VC), forced expiratory volume per one second (FEV_1), inspiratory capacity, functional residual capacity, expiratory and inspiratory reserve volumes, tidal volume, respiration rate, and volume/flow relationships. Clinical spirometers allow for each of the respiratory values to be compared to predicted values based on the person's age, height, and sex, according to various formulae (Kory et al., 1961; Boren et al., 1966 ; Knudson et al., 1983). Although spirometry is unsuitable for the measurement of small, rapid volume changes that occur during speech, the technique is most valuable in providing objective measurement of lung capacities, and as such, provides a reliable means whereby progressive and remitting changes in respiratory function of persons with MS may be monitored.

The kinematic assessment of respiratory function determines airflow volume changes indirectly from displacements of the components of the chest wall, i.e. the rib cage and abdomen. This method of assessment is based on kinematic theory which considers the chest wall to be a two-part system consisting of the rib cage and diaphragm-abdomen, arranged in mechanical parallel (Hixon et al., 1973). As the chest wall and abdomen move, they each displace a volume which, when combined, is equal to that of the lungs (Hixon et al., 1973). This technique involves the simultaneous yet independent recordings of the components of the chest wall during speech (vowel and syllable prolongations, reading, counting, and conversational speech) and nonspeech tasks, thus providing a more comprehensive evaluation of respiratory function. Four main types of kinematic instrumentation are available in research and/or clinical settings: magnetometers (Hixon et al., 1983; Hoit and Hixon, 1986, 1987; Hodge and Putnam-Rochet, 1989; McFarland and Smith, 1992; Solomon and Hixon, 1993; Stathopoulos and Sapienza, 1993); strain-gauge pneumograph systems (Murdoch et al., 1989a, 1989b; Manifold and Murdoch, 1993; Murdoch et al.,1993); mercury strain-gauges (Baken et al.,1979; Cavallo and Baken, 1985); and inductance plethysmography (Lane et al.,1991; Sperry and Klich, 1992; Winkworth et al., 1995).

Respiratory inductance plethysmography, commercially available as the Respitrace (Ambulatory Monitoring Inc.), currently forms the basis of respiratory assessment within the authors' own laboratory. This instrumentation has been found to provide useful information regarding respiratory function in a variety of neurologically disordered populations, including persons with MS. Movements of the rib cage and abdomen during speech breathing are detected through changes in the inductance of a zigzag arrangement of wires inserted into elastic bands, positioned around the rib cage and abdomen. An oscillator produces a frequency-modulated signal which is directed through the wires in the elastic bands. Changes in chest wall circumference during breathing affect the shape, and therefore the conductance of the wires in the elastic bands, resulting in a change in the signal. In addition to providing an effective means of assessing respiratory function, the visual display of the signal output of the Respitrace system may be utilized as a biofeed-back facility for those persons with impairment of co-ordination of the components of the chest wall during speech breathing.

Physiological features of respiratory dysfunction in multiple sclerosis

Investigations of the physiological aspects of respiratory function in persons with MS have involved measures of flow rates, lung volumes, maximal voluntary ventilation, maximal respiratory pressures, and kinematic evaluations of speech breathing. In their early study of dysarthria associated with MS, Darley et al. (1972) identified decreased vital capacities (i.e. < 80% of the normative values for subjects of similar age, sex, and height) in approximately one-third of their MS group. Smeltzer et al. (1988), in a study of 25 patients with MS, identified varying degrees of pulmonary dysfunction depending on the individual's overall level of disability. An ambulatory patient group recorded normal forced vital capacities (FVC), maximal voluntary venti-lation (MVV) values, and maximal expiratory pressures (MEP) (mean > 80% predicted) while these values were reduced in wheelchair-bound patients with upper extremity involvement (mean = 69.4%, 50.4%, 62.6%, predicted, for FVC, MVV, MEP, respectively), and those patients who were bedridden (mean = 38.5%, 31.6%, 36.3%, predicted, for FVC, MVV, MEP, respectively). Expiratory muscle weakness was found to occur most frequently, and with increasing severity, in patients with progressive involvement of the upper extremities. In a more extensive study of respiratory function in MS, however, Smeltzer et al. (1992) failed to record reductions in vital capacity and forced expiratory volume per one second on standardized spirometric assessments in a group of 40 MS subjects who demonstrated a broad range of general motor dysfunction. These MS subjects, however, were found to demonstrate reductions in MVV values (mean = 68%, predicted), peak expiratory flow rates (PEFR) (mean = 71%, predicted), maximal expiratory pressures (PEmax) (mean = 51%, predicted), and maximal inspiratory pressures (PImax) (mean = 74%, predicted). The 12 patients with dysarthria in this study were found to demonstrate significantly reduced maximal expiratory pressures compared to the non-dysarthric speakers. Similar studies of respiratory function in persons with MS have consistently identified abnormal respiratory muscle function in these subjects with a predominance of weakness in the expiratory musculature (Howard et al., 1992; Tantucci et al., 1994; Buyse et al., 1997; Gosselink et al., 1999).

Recently, we assessed the respiratory function of a group of 33 subjects with MS (see Table 4.1 for biographical and clinical details of these subjects) using both spirometric and kinematic techniques. Consistent with the findings of Darley et al. (1972), the MS subjects were found to demonstrate significant reductions in the absolute values for vital capacity compared to the control group, with a corresponding reduction in the mean predicted value for the group (77%), based on normative data from subjects of similar age, sex, and height. Similarly, the 10 dysarthric speakers in the sample were found to exhibit significantly reduced vital capacities compared to the control subjects, with a mean predicted value of 68.5%. As a group, however, the MS subjects did not demonstrate significant reductions in FEV_1, although the 10 dysarthric MS speakers recorded a lower than normal mean predicted value of 70.5% for this parameter.

Kinematic evaluation of respiration revealed abnormal patterns of speech breathing in the MS subjects compared to the control group. During maximum respiratory effort tasks (vowel prolongation, syllable repetition, and counting on a single exhalation), the MS group demonstrated significantly reduced lung volume excursions compared to the control group. The reductions in lung volume excursions on the vowel prolongation and syllable repetition tasks appeared to be due to the significantly elevated lung volume termination values recorded for the MS subjects. During these speech activities, the subjects with MS were initiating speech at a similar lung volume to the control subjects but terminating speech at a higher lung volume than their control counter-parts, i.e. the MS subjects were not utilizing their full lung capacity during the maximum respiratory effort tasks. The bases of the reduced lung volumes recorded by the MS subjects were identified in the analyses of the kinematics of the components of the chest wall which revealed similar significant reductions in rib cage and abdominal excur-sions due to elevated termination levels during maximum respiratory effort tasks. During counting on a single exhalation, the MS subjects were also found to exhibit significantly reduced rib cage excursions.

For conversational speech, however, the MS subjects demonstrated a different pattern of speech breathing compared to that produced on maximum respiratory effort tasks. The lung volume excursions recorded for the MS subjects during conversational speech were found to be significantly increased compared to the control group due to the former subjects initiating speech at significantly higher lung volumes, but at similar termination levels to the controls. The MS subjects, however, were found to demonstrate a similar breathing pattern to their control counterparts during a reading task. Interestingly, when the respiratory patterns of the 10 dysarthric MS speakers were compared with the control group, the former subjects were found to demonstrate similar breathing patterns to this group, except during counting where the rib cage excursions of the MS dysarthric speakers were found to be signifi-cantly reduced. These findings for the subjects with dysarthria most probably reflect the small size of this group, as well as the mild degree of severity of the dysarthric speech disturbance evident in the majority of these subjects. Larger sample sizes of MS persons with varying degrees of severity of dysarthria may well result in differences in speech breathing patterns between MS dysarthric speakers and control subjects.

As inco-ordination of the chest wall components, in the form of rib cage and abdominal paradoxing and slope changes (Murdoch et al., 1993), may contribute to disturbances in the expiratory airflow during speech, the expiratory traces recorded on the Respitrace during the speech tasks were visually inspected to determine the frequency of these abnormal respiratory patterns. While many instances of rib cage and abdominal paradoxing and slope changes were identified during vowel prolongation, syllable repetition, and counting tasks, these aberrations were not found to be significantly more frequent in the breathing patterns of persons with MS when compared to non-neurologically impaired individuals. Furthermore, the group of 10 dysarthric speakers with MS failed to demonstrate a significantly greater frequency of paradoxical movements and slope changes than the control subjects.

Further analyses of speech breathing parameters for the 33 MS subjects revealed that these subjects demonstrated significant impairments in breath control and speaking rate with reductions in the number of syllables per breath (mean = 9.85) and syllables per minute (mean = 157.56) produced during a reading task, compared to the control group (mean = 12.96 syllables per breath; mean = 212.07 syllables per minute). Significant reductions in breath control and speaking rate were also identified in the MS dysarthric speakers (mean = 9.07 syllables per breath; mean = 145.25 syllables per minute).

Subclinical manifestations of respiratory dysfunction in multiple sclerosis

Despite the presence of perceptually normal speech in many persons with MS, there is both perceptual and physiological evidence of subclinical respiratory dysfunction in these persons. Perceptual data supporting the presence of subclinical respiratory impairment in persons with MS have been reported by Hartelius et al. (1993) who found that 16 non-dysarthric MS subjects were significantly impaired on a range of clinical respiratory tasks, compared to control subjects. The respiratory tasks included sniffing, panting, prolongation of /s/, effecting sudden loudness increases on /s/ and /a/, shouting, and producing expiratory pressure at 5 cm H20 for a period of time. Similarly, 20 non-dysarthric MS subjects examined in the authors' own study outlined above, demonstrated significantly greater impairment than control subjects on the respiratory subtests of the FDA relating to respiration at rest and during speech. The MS individuals with perceptually normal speech production were found to demonstrate a mild impairment of respiratory function at rest and during speech.

Physiological evidence of subclinical manifestations of respiratory dysfunction has been identified in individuals with MS in relation to respiratory muscle weakness, abnormal patterns of speech breathing, and reduced vital capacities and speaking rate. Respiratory muscle weakness has been identified following specific tests of respiratory muscle strength in some subjects with MS who did not report any pulmonary symptoms (Smeltzer et al.,1988). These investigators found that some individuals who were wheelchair-bound demonstrated significantly impaired forced vital capacity, maximal voluntary ventilation, and maximal expiratory pressure even though the subjects themselves did not report the presence of respiratory symptoms such as dyspnoea. Similarly, Gosselink et al. (1999) concluded that there was a poor correlation between the degree of muscle weakness and pulmonary function as MS patients with normal or near normal pulmonary function were found to demonstrate respiratory muscle weakness. Furthermore, impaired respiratory muscle function has been found to occur early in the course of the disease, long before clinical symptoms of respiratory dysfunction are manifested (Gosselink et al., 1999).

The analyses of respiratory function in persons with MS, conducted in the authors' laboratory, have identified abnormal patterns of speech breathing in individuals who, at the time of testing, did not exhibit a dysarthric speech disturbance. Specifically, the non-dysarthric MS subjects demonstrated significantly reduced lung, abdominal, and rib cage excursions during maximal effort tasks which were related to corresponding increases in volume termination values. During conversational and reading tasks, however, the non-dysarthric MS subjects were not found to be significantly different to the control subjects. The abnormal speech breathing patterns demonstrated by the non-dysarthric MS subjects during maximal effort tasks may reflect the presence of respiratory muscle weakness that has been identified in persons with MS, particularly in the early stages of the disease (Smeltzer et al., 1992; Gosselink et al., 1999). Such weakness prevents the individual from achieving a normal range of chest wall movement during these types of activities. As conversational speech and reading aloud do not require the same degree of lung volume and respiratory muscle strength, speech breathing patterns for persons with MS remain consistent with those of non-neurologically impaired individuals. Impairments in lung volume excursions in MS subjects with no evidence of dysarthria are consistent with the finding of a significant reduction in the mean vital capacity for these subjects compared to controls. While both clinical and subclinical features of respiratory dysfunction in persons with MS have been identified perceptually and physiologically, the impact of these impairments on speech production in the MS population should be evaluated within the context of other aspects of the speech production mechanism, such as laryngeal, velopharyngeal, and articulatory function.

Summary and conclusions

The evidence to date, relating to laryngeal and respiratory dysfunction in persons with MS, suggests that, both perceptually and physiologically, individuals with MS demonstrate varying degrees of impairment in each of these subsystems of the speech mechanism. Although the high incidence of phonatory disorders perceived to be present in the speech of persons with MS has not yet been confirmed physiologically through group data, due to low subject numbers and mild degree of severity of impairment in the particular MS population investigated, there remains sufficient evidence at an individual level to suggest that abnormalities in vocal fold vibratory patterns and laryngeal aerodynamics are apparent in some cases both clinically and subclinically. Currently, however, there is a body of physiological evidence that confirms the perceptual presence of respiratory dysfunction in persons with MS and this impairment may be recorded in both dysarthric and non-dysarthric speakers with MS.

Ongoing research, however, is essential to investigate laryngeal and respiratory impairment across the range of neurological impairment observed in the MS population.

Chapter 6
Treatment of motor speech disorders in multiple sclerosis

Deborah G Theodoros and Elizabeth C Ward

Introduction

The treatment of the dysarthric speech disturbance in individuals with MS presents an ongoing challenge to speech pathologists to maintain a level of functional communicative independence in their clients against a background of progressive, unpredictable neurological impairment. As a result of the progressive demyelination of the central nervous system, one of the most difficult features of MS affecting the rehabilitation of motor speech disorders is the lack of a single and/or static lesion. The functional communicative status of the individual may change with exacerbations and remissions and will require reassessment after each fluctuation in disease activity (Erickson et al., 1989). Kraft (1998) has suggested that we should 'overrehabilitate' these individuals by teaching them strategies that they can employ during periods of exacerbation. For those persons with a chronically progressive disease process devoid of exacerbations and remissions, ongoing evaluation of communicative function is inherent within a management programme. Underpinning any treatment programme for persons with MS is the awareness that fatigue is the most common problem experienced by persons with MS (Freal et al., 1984) and must be considered in relation to the duration and intensity of treatment.

The importance of addressing the dysarthric disturbance in persons with MS cannot be overstated as the need to maintain functional communication becomes even more important for these individuals with progressive loss of control of physical mobility (Farmakides and Boone, 1960). As it has been found that increasing mobility restriction is associated with an increase in the frequency of communication disorders in persons with MS (Beukelman et al., 1985), it is imperative that intervention is proactive in keeping pace with progressive deterioration of the central nervous system with the aim of maintaining, at the very least, a functional level of communication in individuals with MS. In treating these clients, the clinician is faced with difficult management decisions in relation to the initiation, intensity, and duration of therapy, and the therapeutic approach most appropriate to each client at different stages of the disease. The wide variability of presentation of the dysarthric speech disturbance in persons with MS requires clinicians to be creative and eclectic in their approaches to the management of dysarthria in this population.

An eclectic approach to the treatment of persons with MS and dysarthria may encompass: an early intervention component; therapy to improve and maintain specific motor speech subsystem function and speech intelligibility; a functional communication approach; and, for the more severely impaired individuals, the use of augmentative and alternative communication systems. While all of these components have been developed generically and used for the treatment of dysarthric speech disturbances associated with various neurological impairments, to date, there has been minimal documented research into the treatment of dysarthria specifically associated with multiple sclerosis.

Early intervention

The importance of early intervention in the treatment of dysarthria associated with MS is a recognized and acceptable theoretical principle which, unfortunately, has received minimal clinical application. Rosenbek and LaPointe (1991) advocated early intervention in the treatment of dysarthria associated with slowly progressive diseases to impede the degeneration of speech function. Similarly, Berry (1983) espoused the importance of early referral of patients with other degenerative disorders such as Parkinson's disease, even before the dysarthric speech disturbance becomes apparent, to educate the individual in relation to the possible ensuing speech difficulties, and to instigate therapeutic procedures to retard the effects of the disease process.

A recent study by Hartelius, Wising and Nord (1997) involving an intervention programme based on increasing vocal efficiency and improving contrastive stress in seven dysarthric speakers with MS revealed that factors contributing to an improvement in prosody were easier to develop in those individuals who were in the early stages of the disease and exhibiting a mild dysarthria, than with persons exhibiting a more severe dysarthria and greater severity of neurological involvement. These investigators concluded that early intervention to improve contrastive stress would seem to be more appropriate than addressing this aspect of a motor speech disorder at a later stage in the disease process.

Recent research has provided evidence to suggest that intervention may be appropriate at an even earlier stage of the disease process i.e. before a dysarthric speech disturbance has become apparent. Subclinical manifestations of motor speech dysfunction in persons with MS have been identified in various components of the speech mechanism in non-dysarthric speakers with MS. Hartelius et al. (1993), during a clinical evaluation of motor speech subsystems, identified subclinical manifestations of the disease in the oromotor skills, respiration and phonation of a group of 16 non-dysarthric MS speakers. Specifically, preclinical signs were most apparent in the laryngeal and articulatory subsystems. Similarly, physiological investigations of respiratory function in MS subjects conducted in the authors' own laboratory (see Chapter 5) revealed preclinical evidence of significantly reduced speaking rates as well as abnormal patterns of speech breathing in the form of reduced lung, abdominal, and rib cage excursions during maximal effort speech tasks in non-dysarthric MS speakers compared to normal subjects. Preclinical signs of tongue and lip dysfunction including significantly reduced rates of repetitive tongue movements and decreased lip and tongue strength endurance were also identified in non-dysarthric MS speakers. Furthermore, in the cohort of non-dysarthric MS persons in our study, the Frenchay Dysarthria Assessment (Enderby, 1983) revealed the presence of subclinical manifestations of laryngeal impairment including reduced phonation times, alterations in vocal quality, and decreased pitch and loudness variability compared to normal speakers. Physiologically, 39% of the non-dysarthric MS speakers demonstrated some abnormality in relation to laryngeal aerodynamics and/or vocal fold vibratory patterns.

The presence of dysfunction in the speech production mechanism of persons with MS who perceptually do not demonstrate a dysarthric speech disturbance, highlights the possibility that early assessment and intervention during these preclinical stages may be warranted to provide the individual with strategies to assist in maintaining motor speech function for as long as possible. Such intervention may take the form of individual or group therapy programmes which are community-based and easily accessible on a regular basis.

Specific therapy approaches and techniques

In that MS can affect all subsystems of the speech production mechanism at some stage during the course of the disease, the treatment of a dysarthric speech disturbance in any individual with this condition may involve the use of a number of specific therapy approaches and techniques designed to address impairment in the respiratory, laryngeal, velopharyngeal, and articulatory subsystems. Determining the appropriate treatment approaches and techniques for each dysarthric speaker with MS is contingent upon the type of dysarthria/s and physiological features exhibited by the individual. With changes in the neurological status of the person, these treatment strategies will need to be adjusted accordingly.

Treatment of respiratory dysfunction in MS

The major aims associated with the treatment of respiratory function in individuals with MS include the establishment of adequate breath supply, consistent subglottal pressure, and controlled exhalation during speech. The most common forms of treatment include behavioural, instrumental, and prosthetic management approaches. The specific techniques that may be utilized under these approaches at various times throughout the course of the disease are outlined in Table 6.1. While many of the behavioural and instrumental techniques are the most commonly used techniques for the majority of persons with MS, the prosthetic techniques are more likely to be appropriate for some individuals with MS during periods of exacerbation or for the more severely impaired cases.

Treatment of laryngeal dysfunction and phonatory disorders in MS

Laryngeal subsystem dysfunction due to MS may have a considerable impact on speech intelligibility due to the effects of this impairment on the phonatory, articulatory, and prosodic aspects of speech production (Ramig, 1992). Specifically, laryngeal impairment affects vocal quality, voice-voiceless contrasts, levels and variability of pitch and loudness, and intonation (Ramig and Scherer, 1989). The neurological effects of MS on the laryngeal subsystem of individuals with this disease may result in disorders of vocal fold adduction (hyperadduction or hypoadduction), phonatory instability, and phonatory inco-ordination. Hyperadduction of the vocal folds results in varying degrees of harshness and strain-strangled vocal quality (Aronson, 1985). Where hyperadduction occurs in a patient with MS, management is aimed at reducing the degree of vocal fold adduction and laryngeal resistance to air flow through the glottis and establishing normal vocal fold vibratory patterns. Hypoadduction of the vocal folds results in a reduction of vocal volume, breathiness, hoarseness, and reduced phonation times (Aronson, 1985; Bless, 1988). The treatment of hypoadduction of the vocal folds in persons with MS involves increasing the adduction of the vocal folds through physiologically effortful tasks.

Table 6.1 Specific approaches and techniques for the treatment of respiratory dysfunction in MS

Approaches and techniques	Description	References
A) Behavioural		
Establish and maintain optimal posture	Person supported by pillows and foam supports to obtain and maintain optimal positioning	Netsell and Rosenbek (1985), Rosenbek and LaPointe (1991)
Instruction re normal process of respiration and development of self-monitoring skills	Auditory, visual, and tactile cues (person places hand on abdomen and observes and feels movement of abdomen during inspiration and expiration, monitors exhalation of air auditorially)	Theodoros and Thompson (1998)
Providing abdominal support during exhalation	Push against abdomen during exhalation	Rosenbek and LaPointe (1991)
Pushing, pulling, bearing down activities during speech activities	Push or pull up against stationary object	Prater and Swift (1984)
Inspiratory checking	Involves deep inspiration followed by slow exhalation Makes use of passive recoil pressures of lungs	Netsell and Hixon (1992)
Breath control exercises	Maximum phonation tasks involving vowel prolongation Serial speech tasks of increasing length performed on the one breath Establishing optimal breath groups (number of syllables produced comfortably on one breath)	Moncur and Brackett (1974)
Accent Method	Breathing exercises designed to assist voicing control Emphasis is on transferring respiratory effort to the abdominal region during speech breathing	Kotby (1995)
Breath patterning	Establishing appropriate breath patterns for speech, e.g. rapid intake of air followed by long controlled exhalation Develop ability to 'top up' respiratory supply with catch breaths during speech, pause without inhalation, use variable respiratory patterns	Yorkston et al. (1988)

B) Instrumental

Technique	Description	Reference
U tube manometer	U-shaped thin plastic tubing filled with coloured water and marked with centimetre gradations to indicate the movement of the water. The person blows into one end of tubing and displaces the level of water. For normal speech–need to maintain 5 to 10 cm water for 5 seconds (Netsell and Rosenbek, 1985)	Rosenbek and LaPointe (1991)
Glass and straw system	Glass filled with water with a straw secured to side of glass to a measured depth, e.g. 5 cm. Person required to blow a steady stream of bubbles. When straw positioned to a depth of 5 cm, then person is generating 5 cm respiratory pressure	Hixon, Hawley and Wilson (1982)
Respiratory kinematic feedback	Respitrace system used to display simultaneous but independent movements of the rib cage and abdomen during speech breathing. Useful for improving inco-ordination of the respiratory muscles, respiratory-phonatory timing, and breath control, increasing lung volumes, and promoting abdominal breathing patterns	Murdoch, Sterling and Theodoros (1995) Thompson-Ward, Murdoch and Stokes (1997)

C) Prosthetic

Technique	Description	Reference
Expiratory board or paddle	Board attached to person's chair at the level of the abdominal muscles. Person leans against board to force air from lungs during exhalation in presence of weak abdominal muscles	Rosenbek and LaPointe (1991)
Overhead sling	Person positions arms in overhead sling and pushes down to force expiratory breath from the lungs. Appropriate for severely compromised abdominal musculature and/or for those individuals who remain semi-reclined in bed	Rosenbek and LaPointe (1991)
Abdominal binding or 'girdling'	Elastic bandage or wide leather belt positioned around the abdomen beneath the rib cage to support abdominal musculature and assist with recoil during expiration - Short periods of use only	Rosenbek and LaPointe (1991)

Phonatory instability in MS speakers in the form of glottal fry, diplo-
phonia, vocal tremor, and ventricular phonation may be the result of
neuromuscular abnormalities of the larynx such as perturbations of the
laryngeal musculature, abnormal glottal adduction, oscillation of the
vocal tract tissue, and airflow disturbances (Ramig and Scherer, 1989).
Treatment of phonatory instability is aimed at increasing steadiness and
clarity of phonation. Phonatory inco-ordination involves poor synchro-
nization of phonation with exhalation resulting in delays in voice onset
and offset (Yorkston et al., 1988) as well as inco-ordination between the
laryngeal and articulatory subsystems of the speech mechanism resulting
in impaired production of voice-voiceless contrasts (Kent and Rosenbek,
1982; Weismer, 1984; Ramig and Scherer, 1989; Rosenbek and LaPointe,
1991). In addition, phonatory inco-ordination adversely affects prosodic
aspects of speech due to impairment in the control of a number of
parameters associated with this speech process, e.g. subglottal pressure,
vocal fold tension, pitch and loudness variation, pitch level and duration
of phonation (Hirose and Niimi, 1987; Titze and Durham, 1987; Kent,
1988; Ramig and Scherer, 1989). Specific treatment of phonatory inco-
ordination in MS speakers involves the use of a number of techniques
described in the following sections relating to the management of
prosodic and articulatory disturbances.

The choice of laryngeal treatment techniques is based on the
presenting phonatory disturbance, the type of dysarthria and associated
laryngeal pathophysiology, and the impact of other speech subsystem
dysfunction on phonation. Treatment techniques may vary considerably
within a cohort of persons with MS due to the varying effects of neurological impairment evident in these individuals at different levels of the
central nervous system. Those persons with laryngeal dysfunction due to
a predominately spastic dysarthric speech deficit, associated with hyperadduction of the vocal folds, will require very different techniques to
those individuals who present with laryngeal disturbances associated
with a flaccid dysarthric speech disturbance and hypoadducted vocal
folds. Furthermore, these treatment techniques may need to be
reviewed with exacerbation and progression of the disease. A number of
behavioural, instrumental, and prosthetic techniques may be used in the
treatment of laryngeal dysfunction in persons with MS and are detailed
in Table 6.2.

Treatment of velopharyngeal dysfunction and resonatory
disorders in MS

For those persons with MS who demonstrate bilateral upper motor
neurone pathology or lower motor neurone involvement of the vagus
nerve, dysfunction of the velopharyngeal valving mechanism may occur

Table 6.2 Specific approaches and techniques for the treatment of laryngeal dysfunction and phonatory disorders in MS

Approaches and techniques	Description	References
A) Behavioural		
Techniques to reduce vocal fold adduction	Chewing method	Boone (1977)
	Yawn-sigh technique	
	Gentle voice onsets	
	Oral resonance and projection	
	Phonation at high lung volumes → passive abduction of vocal folds due to downward pull of trachea by lowered diaphragm	Smitheran and Hixon (1981)
Techniques to increase vocal fold adduction	Pushing, pulling, and lifting exercises performed simultaneously with phonation	Froeschels, Kastein and Weiss (1955), Boone (1977), Aronson (1985), Boone and McFarlane (1988)
	Hard glottal attack exercises	
	Postural adjustment of the head (turning head to the affected side to decrease distance between vocal folds)	
	Use of a higher pitch	
	Lee Silverman Voice Treatment (LSVT) Program – designed to increase vocal fold adduction using increased physiological effort associated with deep breathing and the production of a loud voice	Ramig, Bonitati, Lemke and Horii (1994)
Techniques to improve phonatory stability	Breath control exercises - initiation of phonation at the beginning of exhalation	Yorkston et al. (1988)
	Maximum duration vowel phonation exercises	Ramig, Mead and DeSanto (1988)
	Breathing patterning involving frequent inspirations and the production of fewer syllables on expiration	Linebaugh (1983)
	Techniques to enhance phonatory effort and vocal fold adduction (as above)	Ramig and Scherer (1989)

(contd)

Table 6.2 (contd)

Approaches and techniques	Description	References
Techniques to improve phonatory co-ordination	See Tables 6.4 and 6.5 below for specific techniques that are also used in the management of articulatory and prosodic disturbances	
Accent Method	Aims to create an optimal balance between expiration and vocal fold power as well as improved co-ordination between the voice produced at the glottis and the resonating cavities. Abdominal-diaphragmatic breathing simultaneously with accentuated rhythmic phonation at various tempos. Appropriate for treatment of each form of laryngeal dysfunction	Kotby (1995), Fex and Kotby (1995)
B) Instrumental		
Visual feedback of pitch, vocal intensity, and duration	Visipitch Visispeech Speech Viewer	Yorkston et al. (1988) Johnson and Pring (1990) Bougle, Ryalls and Le Dorze (1995)
Visual feedback of respiratory-phonatory co-ordination	Respitrace system (to provide feedback of breath control) in conjunction with Visipitch (feedback of phonation) Strain-gauge respiratory kinematic system in conjunction with a throat accelerometer	Yorkston et al. (1988) Thompson and Murdoch (1995)
Visual feedback of vocal fold movement	Videolaryngoscopy	Bastian (1987)
Visual feedback of air pressure and air flow	Air pressure and air flow transducers coupled to storage oscilloscope	Netsell and Daniel (1979), Simpson, Till and Goff (1988)

Auditory feedback of laryngeal tension	Electromyography (EMG) – use of surface electrodes placed over the cricothyroid region of the larynx to monitor degree of laryngeal tension via auditory feedback	Prosek, Montgomery, Walden, and Schwartz (1978)
C) Prosthetic		
Increase voice intensity	Voice amplifier	Allen (1970)
	Edinburgh Masker – delivers white masking noise to speaker, resulting in an increase in vocal intensity	Adams and Lang (1992)

to varying degrees. As a result, these individuals may exhibit variable hypernasality and nasal air emission during speech production. The treatment of velopharyngeal dysfunction and resonatory disorders in MS dysarthric speakers will be dependent upon the nature and severity of the impairment. Velopharyngeal dysfunction may include either a reduced ability to elevate the soft palate, or intermittent or inappropriate velar opening due to poor coordination. These types of impairment may be related to the predominant dysarthria exhibited by the individual. For example, those persons with a mainly ataxic dysarthria are more likely to exhibit impaired velar coordination compared to individuals with a predominantly spastic or flaccid dysarthria who primarily present with reduced velar elevation. The treatment of a mild degree of velopharyngeal dysfunction and hypernasality may be adequately managed through the use of techniques which focus on improving articulatory function and enhancing oral resonance rather than therapy directed at improving the valving mechanism *per se*. For those cases who present with a mild to moderate degree of hypernasality, the choice of management strategies will depend upon ascertaining the relative severity of involvement in other subsystems of the speech mechanism, determining whether or not the treatment of the velopharynx would enhance function in other subsystems (e.g. respiratory system), and whether or not velopharyngeal function would benefit from treating other components initially (Netsell and Rosenbek, 1985). Severe impairment of velopharyngeal function is often the first priority of intervention as dysfunction of the valving mechanism to this degree can adversely affect respiratory function due to wastage of expiratory air flow and articulatory precision as a result of reduced intraoral pressure. The current behavioural, instrumental, and prosthetic treatment strategies for velopharyngeal dysfunction and hypernasality for all degrees of impairment are outlined in Table 6.3.

Treatment of articulatory disturbances in MS

Treatment strategies employed to remediate articulatory disturbances in persons with dysarthria generally involve techniques to normalize function or reduce impairment of the oral articulators, and to assist the person to compensate for the motor speech impairment. For most individuals with MS, the traditional focus of articulatory treatment has been to establish and maintain compensated speech intelligibility and naturalness of speech production and provide specific articulation therapy. An emphasis on altering muscle tone and strengthening the oral articulators has not usually been a primary focus of therapy in the MS population. Generally, it is considered that little improvement is made in these aspects of muscle function using traditional behavioural techniques and that fatigue and the progressive nature of the disease will tend to override any gains. Kraft (1998), however, suggests that indeed there is a role for resistive exercise for increasing muscle strength in persons with MS. Studies of the effectiveness of resistive exercises for lower leg muscles in mildly and more severely affected individuals with MS have revealed that both of these groups of subjects improved on functional physical activities following resistive muscle exercise (Kraft et al., 1996). Although these findings relate to limb muscles, they do suggest that resistive muscle exercising of the oral articulators should not be readily discounted in persons with MS without further investigation of the possible positive effects of this treatment. For individuals, however, who present with predominantly ataxic dysarthria, treatment techniques designed to address lip, tongue, and jaw dysfunction should focus more specifically on the control and direction of movement of the articulators rather than on improving strength and tone. Specific behavioural and instrumental treatment strategies for the treatment of articulatory disorders are outlined in Table 6.4.

Treatment of prosodic disorders in MS

Prosodic disorders involving the stress patterning, intonation, and rate of speech have been identified in persons with MS. In that prosody contributes significantly to the meaning of an utterance, the treatment of this aspect of speech production should be initiated as early as possible in the intervention programme to maximize speech intelligibility (Yorkston et al., 1988; Rosenbek and LaPointe, 1991). A range of behavioural, instrumental, and prosthetic techniques are available for the management of prosodic disorders in persons with MS (see Table 6.5).

Functional communication approach

For many persons with MS and associated dysarthria, the functional communication approach to treatment will constitute an inherent component of their overall management programme. The basis of this approach is that the individual is assisted to learn to communicate effectively, by whatever means, during everyday activities and social interactions without specifically addressing the speech deficit *per se* (Aten, 1994). The direction the approach takes is determined by the needs and life activities specific to the individual. For persons with a degenerating disorder as in MS, the specific components of a functional communication programme will need to be modified according to the changing communication status of the individual.

Table 6.3 Specific approaches and techniques for the treatment of velopharyngeal dysfunction and resonatory disorders in MS

Approaches and techniques	Description	References
A) Behavioural		
Increase palatal awareness	Palatal massage – The palate is massaged in both the anterior-posterior and medial-lateral directions and elevated during the production of non-nasal sounds. The patient can then be encouraged to elevate the palate away from the finger	Rosenbek and LaPointe (1991)
Use of pressure, icing, brushing or vibration on the velum	Prolonged icing. Pressure to muscle insertion points. Slow and irregular brushing and stroking. De-sensitization of hyper-reflexias of the velar muscles	Dworkin and Johns (1980)
Improving articulation and oral resonance	Oral resonance therapy – (1) Alters tongue position – need to modify high raised back tongue position to reduce nasal resonance (2) Increases jaw widening	Moncur and Brackett (1974)
B) Instrumental		
Nasometer (Kay Elemetrics)	Provides visual feedback of levels of nasalance (ratio of nasal to oral acoustic output) during speech tasks. Displayed as real-time display or bar graphs. Threshold levels of nasalance can be set during therapy	Theodoros and Thompson (1998)
Velograph	Real-time display of velar movement via an oscillograph	Kunzel (1982)
Electromyography (EMG)	Surface electrodes placed under chin, in front of hyoid bone, to record electrical activity from the glossopalatine muscles during oral facilitation procedures and speech task	Draizar (1984)

Accelerometry	Miniature accelerometers attached to the side of the nose and throat detect vibrations of acoustic energy which are displayed on a computer screen or via an oscillograph. Visual feedback to observe nasal/non-nasal contrasts	Stevens, Kalikow and Willemain (1975)
Continuous Positive Airway Pressure (CPAP) therapy	An air pressure flow device delivers positive air pressure to the nasal cavities via a mask. The air pressure provides resistance for the soft palate to work against during speech tasks to increase strength and subsequently reduce hypernasality	Kuehn and Wachtel (1994)

C) Prosthetic

Palatal lift	Designed to partially elevate the palate and allow the lateral pharyngeal walls to move towards the midline and make contact with the velum. Consists of an individually constructed plastic palate (held in position by wires attached to the maxillary teeth), with a hard plastic shelf which projects posteriorly under the soft palate to artificially elevate the velum. Three factors associated with best prognosis for palatal lift: (1) a large and constant velopharyngeal insufficiency (2) fair to good articulation (3) ability to generate subglottal air pressures of 5–10cm H20 for a typical speech effort	Netsell and Daniel (1979), Netsell and Rosenbek (1985), Yorkston et al. (1988)

Table 6.4 Specific approaches and techniques for the treatment of articulatory dysfunction in MS

Approaches and techniques	Description	References
A) Behavioural		
Altering muscle tone	Hypertonia – jaw shaking, chewing method, and progressive relaxation Hypotonia – increasing speaking effort	Boone (1977), McClosky (1977), Rosenbek and LaPointe (1991)
Increasing muscle strength	Isotonic (repetitive movements without resistance) and isometric (movements against resistance) exercises involving lips, tongue and jaw Groups of 5 – 10 repetitions	Rosenbek and LaPointe (1991)
Improving control and direction of movement	Specific speech and nonspeech exercises designed for lip, tongue, and jaw to address co-ordination and direction of movements Movements performed to a set rhythm	Farmakides and Boone (1960)
Articulation therapy	Establish or normalize articulatory targets with progression through short, easy speech units to longer, more demanding utterances	Kearns and Simmons (1988)
Compensated speech intelligibility	Speaker required to make adjustments to speech movement patterns to produce an acceptable speech outcome. Specific speech movements are not taught. Contrastive production drills and Intelligibility drills Voiced-voiceless contrasts – exaggerating aspiration of voiceless sounds, increasing vowel duration before voiced sounds, increasing duration of voiceless plosives compared to voiced cognate.	Yorkston et al. (1988) Rosenbek and LaPointe (1991)

B) Instrumental

Electromyography (EMG)	Biofeedback of muscle tension and strength of articulators	Draizar (1984), Nemec and Cohen (1984), Netsell and Daniel (1979), Rubow, Rosenbek, Collins and Celesia (1984)
Lip and tongue pressure transducers	Biofeedback of lip and tongue strength, endurance and fine motor control	Hinton and Luschei (1992), Robin, Somodi and Luschei (1991), Thompson, Murdoch, Theodoros and Stokes (1996)
Electropalatography	Artificial palate embedded with miniature electrodes. Provides details of the location and the timing of tongue placement against the palate during speech. Electrodes provide visual feedback of tongue patterns and timing	Hardcastle, Gibbon and Jones (1991), Gibbon, Dent and Hardcastle (1993)
Visipitch, air flow and air pressure transducers	Provide feedback of voiced-voiceless distinction. Intensity and duration of sounds, intraoral pressure, air flow	Theodoros and Thompson (1998)

Table 6.5 Specific approaches and techniques for the treatment of prosodic disorders in MS

Approaches and techniques	Description	References
A) Behavioural		
Improving stress patterning	Contrastive stress drills – core sentence of drill consists of two or more components that are differentiated in meaning by varied stress patterns	Rosenbek and LaPointe (1991)
Improving intonation	Establishing and/or improving breath group capacity and pattern	Yorkston et al. (1988)
	Breath group considered unit of prosody	Rosenbek and LaPointe (1991)
	Contrastive intonational drills	Rosenbek and LaPointe (1991)
	Decrease uniformity of breath groups to reduce monotony of pitch	Bellaire, Yorkston and Beukelman (1986)
Rate control	Controlled reading tasks – each word presented one at a time	Rosenbek and LaPointe (1991)
	Speech linked to hand tapping at a predetermined rate	
	Rhythmic cueing – words to be read presented in a rhythmic manner by clinician	Yorkston et al. (1988)
	Stress patterning exercises, appropriate phrasing and breath patterning, use of short phrases	Robertson and Thomson (1984)
B) Instrumental		
Feedback of parameters of stress, intonation and rate (duration, intensity, pitch)	Oscillographic feedback	Caligiuri and Murry (1983), Berry and Goshorn (1983)
	Visipitch	
	Speech Viewer	Bougle et al. (1995)

Rate control	Computerized rhythmic cueing – PACER – Regulates speech rate during reading while allowing for the naturalness of speech to be maintained	Beukelman, Yorkston and Tice (1988)
	Delayed auditory feedback (DAF) – Results in a reduction of speech rate and improvements in vocal intensity and fundamental frequency variability, pause time, and speech intelligibility. Average delay of 50msecs	Hanson and Metter (1980)
C) Prosthetic		
Rate control	Pacing board – Speaker required to place finger in separate slots on a board as individual words are spoken	Helm (1979)
	Alphabet board – Speaker identifies first letter of each word on alphabet board, thus slowing speech rate as letter is located	Beukelman and Yorkston (1978), Crow and Enderby (1989)

Table 6.6 Speaker, listener, and communicative interaction strategies for dysarthria in MS

Strategies and techniques	Description	References
A) Speaker strategies		
Indicate how communication will occur	Speaker points to first letter of a word as spoken	Duffy (1995)
	Listener asked to repeat each word or sentence as soon as completed	
	Listener to ask for clarification as soon as communication not understood.	
Identify the context and topic of conversation	Speaker identifies contextual cues e.g., person's name, food items, animal etc.	Dongilli (1994), Duffy (1995)
	Speaker explicitly identifies the topic of conversation, particularly when changing topics within an interaction e.g., from a list of words	
Modify content and length of utterances	Speaker either simplifies content of utterance or elaborates	Duffy (1995)
	Speaker reduces the use of idiomatic expressions and uses more literal expressions	Duffy (1995)
	Speaker reduces or increases length of utterance depending on degree of severity of dysarthria	Dongilli (1994), Yorkston and Beukelman (1978)
Determine listener comprehension	Speaker maintains eye contact with listener and asks if message has been understood	Duffy (1995)
B) Listener strategies		
Modify physical environment	Reduce noise levels and increase signal-to-noise ratio	Berry and Sanders (1983)
	Avoid poorly lit environments	
	Maintain eye contact, adequate speaker-listener distance	

Develop active listening skills	Listener increases attention to speaker	Duffy (1995)
	Listener notifies speaker of level of comprehension	
C) Interaction strategies		
Maintain eye contact		Duffy (1995)
Determine feedback methods	Immediate or delayed feedback	Duffy (1995), Till and Toye (1988),
	Specific feedback of when and where errors occur	Yorkston et al. (1988)
	Request topic	
	Summarize content and identify missing information	
	Specific gesture indicating lack of understanding	
	Cues to facilitate intelligibility e.g. slow down	

The principles of functional communication therapy, as outlined by Aten (1994), may be readily applied to dysarthric speakers with MS and include: an emphasis on communication rather than speech accuracy; the use of therapy materials directly relevant to the person's communicative needs rather than arbitrary drill exercises; active involvement of the person in a communicative interaction; the use of natural feedback of level of communication efficiency as opposed to a level of speech accuracy; utilizing real-life communication environments or instead, simulated events which focus on information exchanges that are readily generalized; focusing on the person's most efficient and effective mode of communication; the elimination or reduction of inefficient and ineffective communicative behaviours; and increasing the communicative interaction opportunities for the individual and the rate of information exchange.

With this more global approach to the treatment of dysarthria in persons with MS, the individual, in conjunction with the clinician, determines specific strategies to facilitate the communicative interaction. A number of communication-oriented strategies relating to the dysarthric speaker, the listener and the communicative interaction *per se*, have been found to be useful for persons with dysarthria (Duffy, 1995) and are outlined in Table 6.6.

Augmentative and alternative communication (AAC)

An augmentative and alternative communication (AAC) approach to the management of the dysarthric speech disturbance exhibited by persons with MS is generally applied to those individuals who have progressed to the later stages of the disease and demonstrate neurological involvement of multiple levels of the central and peripheral nervous systems. In the most severe cases, speech is no longer functional for communication purposes in any setting while for the less severely impaired individual, augmentative communication systems are utilized to supplement deteriorating verbal communication.

The literature concerning the efficacy of AAC for persons with MS has highlighted the importance of early introduction of AAC for individuals with MS. Delaying the process to a stage where neurological and cognitive dysfunction is pervasive limits the clinician in acquiring the relevant information from the person to establish an appropriate AAC system. In addition, such a state of dysfunction in the MS individual severely limits his/her ability to acquire the skills to effectively utilize the device. Porter (1989), in a study of the assessment and application of AAC techniques to a 35-year-old male with advanced MS stressed the importance of assessment early in the course of the disease to design more appropriate systems by identifying communication needs and determining the appropriate vocabulary, and allowing for time to locate and implement the system which will provide the most independent means of communication. Similarly, earlier intervention with AAC in the case of a 30-year-old woman with MS documented by Honsinger (1989) may have reduced the abnormal adaptive communication behaviours in this case and resulted in a more favourable outcome.

In providing an AAC means of communication to an individual with MS, the clinician is faced with considerable challenges in relation to the assessment of the person's communicative needs and abilities, the identification of the appropriate device, and its implementation and maintenance. Determining the communicative needs of the severely dysarthric MS speaker is often more readily achievable compared to defining similar needs in less severely speech disordered persons with MS due to the differing levels of educational, vocational and social involvement of these clients. In general, the severely dysarthric speakers with MS no longer function within an educational or vocational environment due to physical, communicative, and cognitive restraints. Their communicative needs, therefore, are less extensive than their peers and often limited to conversational interaction. For the less severely speech impaired individuals, however, who may continue to participate in a variety of communication settings, the assessment of communication needs will require greater exploration. Regardless of the level of severity of communication impairment, the communicative needs of each person with MS requiring AAC must be clearly identified and detailed by the clinician to ensure that the individual's quality of life is maximized.

A discussion of particular AAC devices and their applications is beyond the scope of this chapter, and we refer the reader to the extensive AAC literature available (Silverman, 1993). Of principal importance to the present chapter, however, are the key issues specific to persons with MS which must be considered in the AAC decision-making process. An assessment of the abilities of each individual with MS to use an AAC system must consider a number of motor, sensory, speech and language, and cognitive skills which may be significantly impaired in persons with MS. Motor impairment which will affect the manipulation of AAC devices may be apparent to varying degrees in the form of ataxic tremor, reduced balance, muscle weakness, and spasticity (Kraft, 1998). Detailed assessment, therefore, by a physiotherapist and occupational therapist, is an essential component of AAC intervention. Visual deficits occur frequently in this population and are often the initial symptom in 16% to 30% of persons with MS (Beukelman and Mirenda, 1992). The extent of visual deficits in persons with MS consequently may preclude some individuals from using sophisticated visual scanning displays. These may be replaced by auditory scanning systems (Beukelman and Mirenda, 1992). Similarly, printed AAC systems may need to be constructed in large print for the MS population and may be complemented by synthetic speech feedback of the letters or words communicated (Honsinger, 1989; Beukelman and Mirenda, 1992).

For any AAC device, it is important that the person's language skills are adequately assessed to determine the level of language function to be incorporated into the AAC system. Similarly, the cognitive function of persons with MS requires detailed assessment as deficits in short-term memory and abstract conceptualization will impact significantly on new learning in these individuals. Beukelman and Mirenda (1992) propose that AAC systems which build on old skills rather than learning completely new ones will be more successful in this population.

Finally, an important aspect of the implementation of AAC systems for persons with MS is the need to ensure that not only has the individual received adequate experience with the system under supervision of the clinician, but that all other individuals within the person's communicative environment are familiar with, or readily able to participate in, the communicative system (Porter, 1989). Due to the progressive nature of the disease, both the implementation and maintenance of AAC systems require a flexible and immediate response to intervention to address the changing needs of the individual.

Treatment efficacy studies in MS

Despite the range of treatment approaches and techniques that are appropriate for the management of the dysarthric speech disturbance associated with MS, documented treatment efficacy studies are limited. Of the small number of studies reported in the literature, some have focused on the treatment of specific aspects of speech such as prosody, vocal volume, articulation, and breath control while others have addressed specific weakness in respiratory musculature. Recently, the effectiveness of a more global approach to the treatment of MS has been investigated and has demonstrated significant improvements in overall neurological deficits in these individuals, including noticeable improvements in the dysarthric speech disturbance.

The earliest efficacy study of the treatment of the dysarthric speech disturbance in persons with MS was reported by Farmakides and Boone (1960) in a retrospective study of 68 patients who had received two to four weeks of daily individual therapy for 20-30 minutes per session. The specific techniques used included: speaking more loudly, breath control exercises, exercises to increase pitch variation, oral resonance exercises, exaggerated articulation, and tongue exercises emphasising control and direction of movement rather than strength. Eighty-five per cent of these cases demonstrated an improvement in speech based on a broad speech progress rating scale. A later study by Caligiuri and Murry (1983) investigated the effectiveness of visual feedback of parameters such as word duration, vocal intensity, and intraoral pressure associated with target stress in the treatment of prosodic control in a subject with MS who presented with a predominantly ataxic dysarthria. Following nine weeks of treatment, the subject demonstrated improvements in speaking rate, prosodic control, and overall level of speech impairment.

In a recent study by Hartelius, Wising and Nord (1997), seven dysarthric MS speakers were involved in an intervention programme to improve vocal efficiency, contrastive stress, and the effective use of verbal repair strategies. Of the seven persons with dysarthria, two were mildly impaired, four demonstrated a moderate speech disturbance, and one subject was noted to be severely dysarthric. Vocal efficiency tasks focused on posture, relaxed abdominal breathing, deep inhalations and controlled exhalations, starting speech at higher lung volumes to reduce spasticity and phonatory instability, increasing the use of the abdominal muscles to control loudness variation, and specifically designed speech exercises to increase pitch and loudness variability. Techniques to achieve effective signalling of contrastive stress included contrastive stress drills, discussion of stress production, reading tasks with words to be stressed underlined, and self-monitoring of stress production. Efficient verbal repairs were targeted by encouraging the subjects to self-monitor their speech and to employ vocal efficiency and contrastive stress techniques previously taught, in continuous speech. Each session lasted 45 minutes to one hour, with the total time of intervention and number of therapy sessions variable within the group. The results of this study showed that five of the subjects demonstrated increased articulatory precision, vocal accuracy, and naturalness of speech post-treatment. Even those subjects who demonstrated only a small or negative therapy outcome were able to increase their ability to signal stress and make qualitatively superior verbal repairs to a greater extent post-treatment.

Although not specifically involving dysarthric MS speakers, efficacy studies relating to the treatment of respiratory dysfunction in persons with MS have been reported in the literature. The results of these studies by Olgiati et al.(1989) and Smeltzer et al. (1996) have indicated that the strength of expiratory musculature can be improved through specific training techniques, e.g. respiratory muscle training (RMT) using expiratory resistive loads. These findings have important implications for dysarthric speakers with respiratory dysfunction in that the treatment of speech breathing difficulties in these individuals may need to involve targeting the weakness in the expiratory muscles more specifically, before breath control strategies during speech can be effective.

Recently in the literature, a series of studies have documented the effectiveness of a new treatment for persons with MS in the form of brief external applications of pulsed electromagnetic fields (EMF) (Sandyk, 1994a, b, 1995a, b, c, 1996, 1997a, b). Following this treatment, significant improvements in neurological and neuropsychological function including bladder and bowel control, vision, fatigue, gait, balance, mood, sleep, speech and cognitive function were reported. Of particular interest are those studies which have reported improvements in the dysarthric speech disturbance in a number of individuals with MS (Sandyk, 1995a, b, c). In a study of two cases with chronic progressive MS, cerebellar dysfunction, and severe dysarthria, Sandyk (1995c) found that, in both cases, following two treatments of EMF, speech improved in clarity with a reduction in nasal resonance, less slurring, increased volume, and greater fluency of speech production. After the second treatment, the speech in each case was considered to be 80% and 50% improved, respectively. Following a further three treatments, the dysarthria in both cases was reported to have resolved completely. The dysarthric speech disturbance had not recurred after an eight month period during which time the subjects received one treatment per month. Sandyk (1995c) suggested that changes in cerebellar neurotransmitter functions were responsible for the resolution of dysarthria in these cases rather than a process of remyelination. He postulated that EMF stimulation increases the production of gamma-amino butyric acid (GABA) production which is utilized by the cerebellar Purkinje cells as a neurotransmitter. As degenerative diseases of the cerebellum are known to be associated with reductions in cerebro-spinal fluid (CSF) GABA levels, Sandyk (1995c) suggested that this deficiency was possibly responsible for the development of dysarthria. Increasing CSF GABA levels through EMF stimulation, therefore, results in a resolution of the dysarthric speech disturbance. Sandyk (1995c) also recognized that the resolution of dysarthria may be due to an increase in cerebellar 5-HT (serotonin) which has also been found to be deficient in degenerative diseases of the cerebellum. To date, however, the mechanisms by which EMF stimulation improves the dysarthric speech disturbance in MS remain unknown. As the current measures of speech change following EMF stimulation reported in the literature to date are relatively subjective and simplistic, further research is also needed to more thoroughly describe and quantify the perceptual and physiological changes in speech production that occur following this treatment.

Summary and conclusions

The treatment of the dysarthric speech disturbance associated with MS within a context of changing neurological function constitutes a major challenge to the speech clinician. Early intervention and flexible ongoing therapy is essential in this population to reduce the impact of the disease progression and maintain an adequate level of communication. The efficacy of the current treatment for these individuals requires urgent validation with further studies exploring the application of other treatment options. Without such research and evidence of treatment effectiveness, support for ongoing treatment for this population with a degenerative neurological disease, against a background of ever-diminishing health funding, will not be achieved.

PART 2
LANGUAGE DISORDERS IN MULTIPLE SCLEROSIS

Chapter 7
Language disorders in multiple sclerosis

BRUCE E MURDOCH AND JENNIFER B LETHLEAN

Introduction

As evidenced by the topics of chapters presented in Part 1 of this book, research into communication disorders of individuals with multiple sclerosis (MS) has tended to concentrate on the motor aspects of speech rather than the possible language problems resulting from subcortical white matter demyelination. There is disagreement in the literature as to whether language problems are associated with MS. Some researchers have documented the presence of language dysfunction occurring early in the disease course (Friedman et al., 1983), while others have suggested that language difficulties are rare in the MS population (Farmakides and Boone, 1960; Herderschee et al., 1987). Rao (1986) recognized the language disturbances that may occur in MS but commented on the limited published studies devoted to vital components of neuropsychological function such as language abilities. He concluded that either this important function has been ignored by researchers or language disruption is a relatively uncommon clinical symptom of the disease. In a more recently reported series of studies, Lethlean and Murdoch (1993, 1994a, b, 1997) have demonstrated that when sufficiently sensitive language tests are used, individuals with MS can be shown to exhibit language problems, in particular difficulties on tasks which require problem-solving, planning, decision-making and abstract reasoning.

Models of white matter participation in language

A number of researchers have highlighted the importance of subcortical white matter pathways in language processing (Damasio et al., 1982; Naeser et al., 1982; Alexander et al., 1987). In particular, researchers

109

have suggested that the disruption of the cerebral white matter, as might occur in MS, may cause language problems by disconnecting deep brain structures from the language areas of the cerebral cortex (Gordon, 1985; Alexander et al., 1987). Several neuroanatomical models of language processing have indicated the importance of neural white matter pathways connecting subcortical structures such as the basal ganglia and thalamus to the cortical language areas in language processing (Crosson, 1985; Alexander et al., 1987; Wallesch and Papagno, 1988). Assuming that white matter pathways in the subcortical region do play an important role in language processing as suggested by the neuroanatomical models, it could be predicted that damage to subcortical white matter pathways in neurological diseases such as MS would result in language impairment. Damasio et al. (1982) emphasized the region of the anterior limb of the internal capsule, which contains major fibre systems including projections from the frontal cortex to the pons; auditory cortex to the head of the caudate nucleus; motor thalamus to the frontal premotor cortex; head of the caudate nucleus to the pallidum; and medio-dorsal thalamus to the prefrontal cortex as potentially important in language processing. For example, Damasio et al. (1982) reported that their subjects exhibited disturbed auditory comprehension and paraphasic errors in spontaneous speech as a result of lesions in the anterior limb of the internal capsule. On the basis of their results, Damasio et al. (1982) postulated that the subcortical aphasic deficits resulted from either a disconnection of important white matter pathways, secondary damage to grey matter neuronal operations, or a combination of the two.

Alexander et al. (1987) regarded white matter pathway lesions as a critical prerequisite to language dysfunction. They developed a detailed schematic outline of clinico-anatomical relationships between subcortical lesions with white matter extensions and aphasic disturbances. Anterior, extra-anterior, anterior superior and superior posterior periventricular white matter lesions, as well as extensions in the temporal isthmus, insular cortex or external capsule or some combination of lesions in these areas were most likely to lead to language disturbances (Alexander et al., 1987). For example, when lesions extend laterally and superiorly from the putamen, the external and extreme capsules and/or the arcuate fasciculus can be disturbed. As a result of this pathway disruption, language disturbances including paraphasic errors in repetition would be expected.

Neuroanatomically, the connectivity of cortical and subcortical structures is provided by subcortical white matter pathways. Rather than proposing a single cortical or subcortical structure as exclusively responsible for a particular language process, researchers have suggested that the white matter pathways are critical for enabling cortical and subcortical structures to work together in a linked communicative system (Lieberman et al., 1986; Wallesch and Papagno, 1988; Robin and Schienberg, 1990). Therefore, damage anywhere in the circuitry of pathways may result in abnormal balances of inhibitory and excitatory influences and in this way impair language processing (Crosson, 1985; Robin and Schienberg, 1990). Moreover, lesions in the corona radiata (containing bundles of cortico-projectional and thalamo-cortical fibres subadjacent to the cortex), and the internal capsule (containing projection fibres which connect auditory, parietal and occipital cortical areas and subcortical nuclei) have been reported as leading to similar language deficits as damage of the pathway endpoint, i.e. the cortex (Hyman and Tranel, 1989). Various models of subcortical participation in language are discussed further in Chapter 9.

Language disorders in multiple sclerosis

Despite a theoretical consideration of the importance of connectivity between the cortical and subcortical structures outlined in various neuroanatomical models of language processing, few studies have tested these models by considering the language abilities of individuals with neurological diseases affecting primarily the white matter of the brain. There is a paucity of studies that adequately document the language abilities of persons with multiple sclerosis.

Evidence from multiple sclerosis case studies

Documentation of the presence of language deficits in the MS population has consisted primarily of descriptions of individual MS cases with severe communication difficulties. Few researchers, however, have presented group studies considering language function in MS. Single case studies of subjects with MS have provided evidence for the presence of a language disorder which may be associated with this disease (Friedman et al., 1983; Day et al., 1987; Achiron et al., 1992). In fact, a variety of language problems have been documented in MS subjects, probably reflecting the variable nature of the disease. Individuals with MS have been reported to present with motor aphasia (Olmos-Lau et al., 1977), global aphasia (Friedman et al., 1983), and a 'fluent' language disorder with alexia and agraphia (Day et al., 1987).

Olmos-Lau et al. (1977) documented a case of a 17-year-old woman's development of motor aphasia during a second episode of MS. Her speech was characterized by absent spontaneous speech, paraphasias in naming and repetition, intact auditory comprehension, preservation of written language and orofacial apraxia.

Friedman et al. (1983) described a case of global aphasia in a 32-year-old woman with MS. The case's speech profile revealed non-fluent language production, severely impaired repetition, naming, reading and writing, and poor comprehension of simple commands. A computerized tomographic (CT) scan at this time revealed white matter plaques in the left periventricular region large enough to interrupt all language pathways including connections from Broca's and Wernicke's areas as well as the arcuate fasciculus. A few months later the subject improved and a year later presented with mild anomia and intact comprehension. However, repetition for long sentences remained slightly affected and her handwriting was poor and agrammatical.

A case report of alexia with agraphia in MS has been described in the literature (Day et al., 1987). This 34-year-old woman presented with a jargonic fluent aphasia, which resolved to the presence of mild language deficits including dysnomia, mildly impaired comprehension and repetition and persistent alexia and agraphia. According to Day et al. (1987), the white matter lesion on the CT scan responsible for the aphasic deficits, alexia and agraphia, was appropriately placed to cause a disconnection of the visual cortex from Wernicke's area and the angular gyrus.

Achiron et al. (1992) described two subjects with a relapsing-remitting disease course who presented with acute onset of severe non-fluent aphasia correlating respectively with large plaques in the left frontal region and the left centrum semiovale as identified by magnetic resonance imaging (MRI). It was suggested that the plaques were sufficiently large enough to disrupt commissural, association and projection fibres in the dominant fronto-temporal region, thus causing motor aphasia.

Evidence from multiple sclerosis group studies

Neuropsychological subtests

Research into the language abilities of groups of MS subjects has primarily been limited to studies that have utilized neuropsychological assessments rather than tests designed specifically to determine linguistic abilities. This has resulted in varied reports concerning the presence or absence of linguistic deficits in MS, with both intact and impaired language abilities having been identified by researchers using language subtests of neuropsychological batteries (see Table 7.1). Language subtests incorporated into neuropsychological assessment batteries are designed to access only basic, functional language abilities but may fail to identify complex linguistic performances of individuals with MS. In fact, performance by MS subjects on restricted language assessments may mask the presence of high-level language difficulties, which may be identified on more complex linguistic tasks. Consequently, studies suggesting linguistic integrity in MS have been based on limited language assessment regimens. Discrepancies in the literature as to whether subjects with MS present with linguistic disturbances may therefore be attributed, in part, to the use of insufficiently sensitive language assessments which may fail to detect 'high-level' language problems.

Neuropsychologists primarily interested in cognition and memory in MS have included language subtests such as naming, verbal fluency, spelling, reading and writing in their investigations. A list of these studies appears in Table 7.1. A number of researchers have documented word-finding difficulties in both chronically progressive and relapsing-remitting MS groups on naming tasks including the Boston Naming Test (BNT), the abbreviated BNT, the Graded Naming Test and other unspecified tests of naming (Jambor, 1969; Caine et al., 1986; Beatty et al., 1990). Other studies, however, have reported intact naming abilities in MS groups (Pozzilli, Passafiume et al., 1991; Ron et al., 1991). Reduced speed of lexical access is another linguistic deficit which has been inconsistently identified in MS groups. This finding is indicated by the reported varied performances of individuals with MS on word fluency tasks (Heaton et al., 1985; FitzGerald et al., 1987; Anzola et al., 1990) and on verbal subtests of the Wechsler Adult Intelligence Scale (WAIS) (Jambor, 1969; Callanan et al., 1989). A majority of studies have reported competent reading, writing and spelling skills and relatively intact comprehension abilities in MS groups (see Table 7.1).

Aphasia test batteries

Language assessments designed to test individuals with aphasia following a cerebrovascular accident have also been employed in MS group studies (Heaton et al., 1985; FitzGerald et al., 1987; Franklin et al., 1988; Wallace and Holmes, 1993). Heaton et al. (1985) used the Aphasia Screening Test (AST) to compare 57 relapsing-remitting and 43 chronically progressive MS subjects with a control group. The chronically progressive MS subjects were found to make significantly more errors on the AST than both the relapsing-remitting and control groups, whereas the relapsing-remitting subjects and the control group performed similarly.

Franklin et al. (1988) assessed 60 subjects with chronically progressive MS using the Multilingual Aphasia Examination and the subtest of commands with auditory sequencing from the Western Aphasia Battery. The authors found that, as a group, the MS subjects' receptive and expressive language skills were not significantly different from the control group. Further examination of the data revealed that 20% of the MS subjects were impaired on visual naming, 23% on tests of oral comprehension of words and phrases and 18% on tests of verbal fluency.

Table 7.1 The results of group studies investigating language abilities in subjects with multiple sclerosis

Task	Researchers	n(*)	Findings
WAIS verbal Subtests	Callanan et al. (1989)	48 (unspec)	intact
	Ivnik (1978)	14 (unspec)	intact
	Jambor (1969)	43 (unspec)	impaired
	Klonoff et al. (1991)	86(RR)	intact
	Lyon-Caen et al. (1986)	30(RR)	intact
	Peyser et al. (1980)	55(unspec)	impaired
	Rao et al. (1985)	47(CP)	impaired
	Rao et al. (1991)	19(CP) 39(RR) 42(CS)	impaired
	Van den Burg et al. (1987)	19(RR)	intact
Comprehension	Anzola et al. (1990)	41(RR)	intact
	Huber et al. (1987)	32(unspec)	intact
Reading	Jambor (1969)	43(unspec)	intact
	Rao et al. (1991)	19(CP) 39(RR) 42(CS)	intact
	Jambor (1969)	43(unspec)	impaired
	Callanan et al. (1989)	48(unspec)	intact
Writing	Jennekens-Schinkel, Laboyrie et al. (1990)	20(CP) 13 (RR)	intact
	Jennekens-Schinkel, Lanser et al. (1990)	19(CP) 20(RR)	intact
	Jennekens-Schinkel, Laboyrie et al. (1990)	20(CP) 13 (RR)	intact
Spelling	Jennekens-Schinkel, Lanser et al. (1990)	19(CP) 20(RR)	intact
	Jambor (1969)	43(unspec)	intact

Note: n = number of subjects; * = disease course; WAIS = Wechsler Adult Intelligence Scale; CP = chronically progressive; RR = relapsing-remitting; unspec = unspecified; CS = chronic stable.

FitzGerald et al. (1987) assessed 20 MS subjects using subtests of the Neurosensory Centre Comprehensive Examination for Aphasia (Spreen and Benton, 1969) and the Wiig-Semel Test of Linguistic Concepts (Wiig and Semel, 1974). More than 50% of the subjects performed at a lower than normal level of functioning on subtests of tactile naming, word fluency, sentence construction, writing to dictation, and articulation. Poor comprehension of logico-grammatical constructions was also documented. Subtests other than word fluency and sentence construction were regarded as influenced by sensory and motor problems.

Although no typical aphasic syndrome was identified in the MS group, the group's language profile appeared to reflect semantic or lexical impairments.

More recently, Wallace and Holmes (1993) identified an MS group's cognitive/linguistic deficits on the Arizona Battery for Communication Disorders. When compared to a control group, the MS subjects attained relatively lower scores on the linguistic subtests assessing object description, generative naming, concept definition, generative writing and picture description abilities. Further research using a larger sample of MS subjects was recommended by Wallace and Holmes (1993) because their MS group only consisted of four individuals with a chronic progressive disease course.

High-level language batteries

Despite the documentation of studies hinting at the presence of linguistic impairment in MS, the majority of researchers have provided inadequate information to enable valid description of a characteristic pattern of language breakdown associated with the disease. As indicated earlier, in the majority of studies, the language tests which have been used are not sufficiently sensitive to detect potential high-level language problems and may be confounded by MS subjects' sensory and motor deficits. Neuropsychological assessments including tests of naming, verbal fluency and verbal subtests of the WAIS fail to incorporate measures of high-level language requiring comprehension of complex commands, interpretation of figurative language, inferential reasoning and high-level verbal explanation abilities. While standardized aphasia assessments may assess the gross language abilities of MS groups, they fail to detect more subtle linguistic impairment. Therefore, there exists a need for more specific assessment of high-level language abilities in the MS population using tests specifically developed for that purpose so as to describe fully the proposed language disorder.

The most extensive study reported to date that has utilized a comprehensive battery of specific linguistic tests to investigate the language abilities of persons with MS is that conducted by Lethlean and Murdoch (1993). Since the publication of our original report in 1993, we have extended our study to include a further 43 subjects with MS. Consequently, the remainder of this chapter will focus on providing a synthesis of the findings of the expanded study, which until this time has not been published.

The subjects examined in our expanded study were 60 individuals with a diagnosis of definite MS. The diagnosis was made by a neurologist on the basis of a combination of neuroradiological and clinical signs.

None of the subjects included in the study had a history of speech or language disorder prior to the onset of MS symptoms (see Chapter 1). Likewise, none of the subjects had any history of dementia, cerebrovascular accident or co-existing neurological disease other than MS. English was the primary language of all those included. Sixty non-neurologically impaired individuals matched for age, sex and level of education served as controls.

The personal and medical details of the 60 subjects with MS involved in the expanded study appear in Tables 7.2 (chronically progressive subjects) and 7.3 (relapsing-remitting subjects). The subject group comprised 21 (35%) males and 39 (65%) females. The average age of the total sample of MS subjects was 49 ± 12 years, with ages ranging from 26 to 76 years. Thirty-two subjects (53%) were classified as having a chronically progressive disease course, while 28 (47%) exhibited a relapsing-remitting disease course.

Subjects included in the study presented at varying stages of the disease. The mean length of illness since the first MS symptoms occurred was 16 ± 11 years ranging from 1 to 53 years. The average age at which first symptoms occurred was 32 ± 10 years ranging from 16 to 64 years, and the average age at diagnosis was 38 ± 11 years, ranging from 20 to 52 years. Fifty-two subjects (87%) were living at home and the remaining eight subjects (13%) were in institutionalized care at the time of assessment (see Tables 7.2 and 7.3). The MS group included subjects with a range of physical disabilities ranging from being wheelchair dependent to fully mobile. Only six subjects had visual disturbances extensive enough to interfere with language testing.

The subjects were administered a battery of tests designed to evaluate a range of language functions including high-level language function. The test battery included the Neurosensory Centre Comprehensive Examination for Aphasia (NCCEA) (Spreen and Benton, 1969), the Boston Naming Test (BNT) (Kaplan et al., 1983), the Wiig-Semel Test of Linguistic Concepts (WST) (Wiig and Semel, 1974), the Test of Language Competence (TLC) (Wiig and Secord, 1985), and The Word Test (TWT) (Jorgensen et al., 1981). Each subject completed the assessments over two to three sessions and the maximum length of a testing session was one and a half hours. Testing was discontinued and completed in a subsequent session if the subject became fatigued and all language tests were carried out under standard conditions in constant and quiet surroundings.

The NCCEA was included in the test battery as it provides a comprehensive test of language abilities. Considering that language problems were anticipated in the MS subjects the NCCEA was considered the most appropriate standardized test to administer to this population. The

NCCEA consists of 20 subtests of language performance and four subtests of visual and tactile function. The 20 language subtests assess comprehension and expression of language, retention of verbal information, and reading and writing abilities. Each subtest of the NCCEA has been standardized according to age and educational level and normed according to three populations: normal adults, aphasic adults and non-aphasic brain-damaged adults. Therefore, the normative data allows for comparison of language function according to each subtest as well as overall language performance.

Fifty-nine MS subjects were administered the NCCEA and completed subtests 1–10 and subtest 20. Subject 48 refused to be tested with the NCCEA. Only 53 subjects completed subtest 11 (Token Test) as the remaining six subjects (subjects 4, 8, 15, 23, 32 and 59) did not have adequate visual acuity and motor abilities to perform the tasks required by this examination. Five subjects (subjects 4, 8, 15, 23 and 32) were unable to attempt subtests 12, 13, 14 and 15 (reading subtests) because of their visual disturbances. The writing assessments (subtests 16 to 19) were not completed by 15 subjects (subjects 1, 2, 4, 5, 6, 8, 9, 15, 17, 23, 24, 25, 27, 32 and 60) because their motor or visual impairments were too severe to enable them to write. For each subject, the NCCEA was administered and scored according to the standard procedure described by Spreen and Benton (1969).

The BNT was incorporated in the language assessment because it is reported to detect mild word retrieval problems (LaBarge et al., 1986). Guilford and Nawojczyk (1988) validated the BNT as a sensitive test of word finding by comparing it to the standardized Test of Word Finding (TOWF) (German, 1986). Results indicated that performance on the BNT correlated highly with scores achieved on the TOWF and the researchers concluded that the BNT provides a reliable measure of confrontation naming (Guilford and Nawojczyk, 1988). All subjects completed this task.

The WST evaluates the comprehension of 50 linguistic concepts requiring logical operations. This test required each subject to answer syntactically and semantically complex yes/no questions, including comparative, passive, temporal, spatial and familial relationship items. All 60 MS subjects were able to complete this assessment.

The TLC uses formats that probe divergent production, cognitive-linguistic flexibility and planning for production. The tasks included require problem-solving, planning and decision-making and/or alternative solutions or responses to the same linguistic input. The tasks included in the TLC involve interpretation of ambiguous sentences, making inferences, recreating sentences, and interpretation of figurative language. It was considered that these tasks reflect 'high-level' language

Table 7.2 Summary of chronically progressive multiple sclerosis subject characteristics

Subject number	Sex	Age#	Education#	Age# at first symptoms	Age# at diagnosis	Duration# of disease	Medications*	Physical status	Visual disturbances	Residence
1	M	44	15	33	37	11	Lioresal (Baclofen), Piroxicane (Feldene)	WC	–	I
2	M	61	15	42	42	19	Lioresal (Baclofen)	WC	–	H
3	M	44	14	27	34	17	None	WC	–	H
4	M	44	11	36	36	8	Lioresal (Baclofen)	WC	+b	H
5	F	31	11	20	22	11	Lioresal (Baclofen), Imipramine (Tofranil), Phenytoin sodium (Dilantin)	WC	–	H
6	F	43	10	26	28	17	Diazepam (Valium)	WC	–	I
7	F	67	12	52	52	15	Imipramine (Tofranil)	WC	–	H
8	F	32	13	23	29	9	Lioresal (Baclofen)	WC	+b	H
9	F	28	17	18	20	10	None	WC	–	H
10	F	42	10	28	29	14	Nortriptyline (Allegron)	WC	–	H
11	F	60	12	48	50	12	None	IM	–	H
12	F	48	12	22	22	26	Carbamazepine (Tegretol)	IM	–	H
13	F	61	12	20	24	41	None	WC	–	H
14	F	49	12	38	48	11	None	IM	–	H
15	F	63	12	61	62	2	Lioresal (Baclofen)	WC	+b	H
16	F	76	10	42	42	34	Propantheline bromide (Probanthine)	WC	–	H
17	F	45	12	17	31	28	Lioresal (Baclofen), Prednisone, Clonazepam (Rivotril)	WC	–	H

No.	Sex						Medication	Mobility	Visual	Residence
18	F	60	8	35	45	25	Diflusinal (Voltarin)	WC	–	H
19	F	43	10	25	30	18	None	WC	–	H
20	M	57	10	21	39	36	None	IM	–	H
21	M	41	10	26	40	15	None	WC	–	H
22	M	69	12	16	53	53	None	IM	–	H
23	F	51	16	40	41	11	Dantrolene sodium (Dantrium)	WC	+b	I
24	F	59	10	19	26	40	Carbamazepine (Tegretol)	WC	–	H
25	F	65	14	64	64	1	Dantrolene sodium (Dantrium), Lioresal (Baclofen), Temazepam (Euhypnos), Piroxicane (Feldene)	WC	–	I
26	F	47	6	37	42	10	None	IM	–	H
27	F	48	10	29	31	19	Lioresal (Baclofen)	WC	–	I
28	M	40	12	23	27	17	Lioresal (Baclofen)	WC	–	H
29	M	50	17	49	50	1	Clonazepam (Rivotril), Fluoxetine (Prozac)	IM	–	H
30	M	64	14	32	62	32	None	WC	–	H
31	M	62	15	34	39	28	Diazepam (Valium), Quinine sulphate (Quinet)	WC	–	H
32	M	71	10	40	65	31	Carbamazepine (Tegretol), Propantheline bromide	WC	+b	I

Note: # = reported in years; * = drug names in brackets represent trade names; M = male; F = female; IM = independently mobile; WC = wheelchair dependent; H = home; I = institution; + = present; – = absent; a = minor visual disturbances; b = significant visual disturbances interfering with language tasks.

Table 7.3 Summary of relapsing-remitting multiple sclerosis subject characteristics

Subject number	Sex	Age#	Education#	Age# at first symptoms	Age# at diagnosis	Duration# of disease	Medications*	Physical status	Visual disturbances	Residence
33	M	46	11	33	39	13	Lioresal (Baclofen)	IM	+[a]	H
34	M	64	10	38	47	26	Lioresal (Baclofen)	WC	+[a]	H
35	M	35	12	32	33	3	None	IM	–	H
36	M	48	10	20	20	28	Lioresal (Baclofen), Amitriptyline (Tryptanol)	WC	–	H
37	M	43	16	37	41	6	Dothiepin (Prothiaden)	WC	–	I
38	F	51	12	35	46	16	Lioresal (Baclofen), Carbamazepine (Tegretol)	IM	–	H
39	F	51	10	38	48	13	Diazepam (Valium), Prochlorperazine (Stemetil)	IM	–	H
40	F	25	10	25	25	1	Lioresal (Baclofen), Nortriptyline (Allegron)	IM	–	H
41	F	41	10	36	39	5	None	IM	–	H
42	F	36	10	22	23	14	None	IM	–	H
43	F	55	10	50	54	5	None	IM	–	H
44	F	63	12	22	28	41	None	IM	–	H
45	F	64	10	39	49	25	None	IM	–	H
46	F	49	12	36	47	13	None	IM	–	H
47	F	35	10	28	35	7	None	IM	–	H
48	F	40	12	31	39	9	Amitriptyline (Tryptanol)	IM	–	H
49	M	42	10	34	34	8	None	WC	–	H
50	M	38	14	37	38	1	Amitriptyline (Tryptanol)	IM	–	H
51	F	36	15	26	31	10	None	IM	–	H

							Drugs			
52	F	45	14	27	30	18	Lioresal (Baclofen), Nitrofurantoin (Macrodantin), Clonazepam (Rivotril), Penthienate (Monodral), Imipramine (Tofranil)	IM	–	H
53	F	48	12	37	40	11	None	IM	–	H
54	F	61	12	55	56	6	Lioresal (Baclofen), Nitrofurantoin (Macrodantin), Diflusinal (Voltarin), Trimipramine (Surmontil)	IM	–	H
55	F	28	15	22	23	6	None	IM	–	H
56	F	33	10	23	26	10	Lioresal (Baclofen), Azathioprine (Imuran), Penthienate (Monodral)	IM	–	H
57	F	45	10	41	42	4	None	IM	–	H
58	M	49	12	43	43	6	None	IM	–	H
59	M	27	15	25	25	2	Lioresal (Baclofen), Phenytoin sodium (Dilantin), Penthienate (Monodral)	WC	+[b]	H
60	F	66	10	30	40	36	None	WC	–	I

Note: # = reported in years; * = drug names in brackets represent trade names; M = male; F = female; IM = independently mobile; WC = wheelchair dependent; I = institution; H = home; + = present; – = absent; a = minor visual disturbances; b = significant visual disturbances interfering with language tasks.

abilities because they entail the use of varied areas of language and extensive cognitive processing. Five subjects were unable to complete subtest 2 (Making Inferences) and one subject was unable to complete subtest 4 (Understanding Metaphoric Expressions) because of their visual problems and resulting reading difficulties. All subjects were presented with both visual and auditory input for all subtests. For example, in subtest 1 (Understanding Ambiguous Sentences) the MS subjects were presented with the sentence in the written form and then the sentence was read out by the examiner. The sentence was then repeated several times if required by the subject.

Although TWT was developed for school-aged children, it was included in the test battery as it provides an indication of the subjects' abilities to recognize and express the critical semantic attributes of their lexicon through the processes of categorizing, defining, verbal reasoning and choosing appropriate words. TWT is composed of six tasks assessing areas of expressive language, namely, associations, synonyms, semantic absurdities, definitions and multiple definitions. All 60 MS subjects completed the six tasks of TWT.

The results of the language assessments administered showed that, as a group, the subjects with MS performed significantly below the control group on measures of high-level language abilities including naming, the comprehension of concepts requiring logico-grammatical operations, repetition of sentences, word fluency, and subtests requiring verbal explanation, verbal reasoning, reconstruction of sentences, definitions of words, and interpretation of absurdities, ambiguities and metaphors. Relative preservation of reading and writing abilities, where sensory and motor abilities allowed completion of the subtests, was also noted in the MS group.

Researchers have recognized that the assessment of language abilities in the MS population is difficult because sensory and motor disturbances may interfere with an MS subject's ability to complete some language tests (FitzGerald et al., 1987). In our expanded study, however, the majority of the language assessments that were incorporated in the test battery did not require maximal motor and sensory abilities. Those subjects who did not have the motor abilities to complete the NCCEA subtests such as the Token Test and the writing assessments, nor optimal visual acuity to complete tasks requiring extensive reading such as the Making Inferences subtest of the TLC, were not included in the statistical comparisons. Consequently, most of the language deficits observed in the MS subjects in our study, except for poor performance on the Tactile Naming subtests of the NCCEA (which may be attributed to motor and sensory impairments), were not the outcome of either motor or sensory difficulties.

Further, dysarthric speech, a symptom often associated with MS, may influence speech intelligibility considerably and interfere with verbal explanation tasks. In our expanded study, however, the influence of dysarthria cannot account for the language difficulties noted in the MS group. Although some individuals presented with perceptual dysarthric symptoms including imprecise articulation and slow rates of speech, all the subjects had intelligible speech in conversation, as judged by a qualified speech/language pathologist. In addition, they were also found to achieve maximum scores on the articulation subtest of the NCCEA (subtest 20) composed of single-word repetition tasks. Subjects with a mild to moderate dysarthria were not disadvantaged on verbal expressive tasks as they were encouraged to complete the language tasks, with the exception of the NCCEA word fluency (subtest 8) and sentence construction (subtest 9) tasks, without time constraints.

It has been suggested by Lethlean and Murdoch (1993) that in previous studies, limited gross measures of language not assessing high-level language abilities may have failed to detect language deficits in groups of MS subjects. In our expanded study, however, the NCCEA revealed that, as a group, the MS subjects performed significantly below the controls on subtests including Description of Use, Sentence Repetition, Reversal of Digits and Word Fluency. While statistically significant differences were identified on the Description of Use and Reversal of Digits subtests it is suggested that the clinical meaningfulness of the differences between the MS group and control group means is questionable. For example, the difference between means for the Description of Use subtest was less than one item.

While the majority of the MS subjects in our expanded study were able to name simple objects as assessed on the Visual Naming subtest of the NCCEA, this assessment was not sensitive enough to detect the naming deficits which were identified in the MS group with a more in-depth assessment of naming. Subtests of the NCCEA assessing Sentence Repetition and Word Fluency abilities appeared to be more sensitive measures of linguistic dysfunction in the MS group. Relatively poor performance by the MS subjects on the Sentence Repetition task when compared to the control group, however, may be attributed to compromised short-term recall memory abilities. Memory difficulty has been described as the most common cognitive complaint in MS (Mahler, 1992) and many studies in the literature have indicated that subjects with MS may present with deficits in recall memory (Jambor, 1969; Rao et al., 1985; Caine et al., 1986; Litvan et al., 1988; Minden et al., 1990). Indeed, the influence of memory dysfunction on language tasks, such as those tasks included in the present study, is an area of research that requires further study.

Our findings support those of previous research documenting the presence of verbal fluency deficits in the MS population (e.g. Beatty et al., 1988). As a group, our MS subjects presented with a significantly lower score on the Word Fluency subtest of the NCCEA relative to the control subjects. Variable performance of the subjects within the MS group on the Word Fluency task was apparent, however, when considering individual cases. Some individual MS subjects, irrespective of disease course, were found to produce fewer words than their controls when asked for words beginning with a specified letter, whereas other MS subjects performed better on this task than their matched controls. Previous research studies have also found that MS subjects with both relapsing-remitting and chronically progressive disease courses perform more poorly on verbal fluency tasks than control subjects (e.g. Rao et al., 1991), whereas others have reported that MS subjects, as a group, perform within normal limits on verbal fluency tasks (e.g. Anzola et al., 1990). It is suggested that discrepancies in the literature reporting the presence or absence of word fluency deficits in the MS population may be attributed to the MS subject selection criteria used by the various research groups. It is possible, for example, that inclusion of subjects with variable forms of the disease may mask or enhance the presence of word fluency deficits in the heterogeneous MS group.

Impaired verbal fluency has been regarded as indicative of a disruption of semantic knowledge structure or impaired retrieval of words from semantic memory (Martin and Fedio, 1983; Obler et al., 1986; Butters et al., 1987; Flicker et al., 1987; Troster et al., 1989). If, in fact, word fluency does test the structure or the retrieval process of the semantic system, then the MS subjects' poor performance on this task in the present study may be indicative of a semantic impairment. According to Kennedy and Murdoch (1990), however, it is important not to base an individual's semantic or lexical abilities on the assessment of word fluency alone as the nature of the deficit underlying the disordered performance can only be speculated on. Impaired initiative and spontaneity, impaired working memory and attentional difficulties are all extralinguistic factors which may interfere with the speed and efficiency of completing a word fluency task (Chertkow and Bub, 1990).

Although the MS subjects in our expanded study were able to name simple objects on the NCCEA, the MS group attained BNT scores significantly below the control mean. The MS subjects, as a group, also performed in the impaired range according to Nicholas et al.'s (1989) normative criteria of a score of 48 or less; however, 34 (77%) individuals within the MS group attained naming scores within the normal range, that is, a score above 48. It is suggested that the MS subjects' significantly poor group performance on the BNT relative to controls reflected a subgroup of 26 (23%) naming impaired individuals who presented with word-finding difficulties.

Word-finding deficits in the MS population have also been identified by researchers who have incorporated naming tests in their assessment of MS individuals, whereas other authors have suggested that MS subjects present with intact naming. Blackwood et al. (1991) assessed 48 MS subjects on the BNT and found that the subjects, as a group, scored within normal limits. Further examination of individual performances on the naming tasks revealed a subset of four individuals with semantic-lexical difficulties (Blackwood et al., 1991). On the basis of Blackwood et al.'s (1991) findings and the results of our own expanded study, it is suggested that not all people with MS present with naming difficulties. However, there seems to be a subset of MS individuals who do have problems with naming tasks.

Factors such as differences in subject selection criteria (e.g. differences in disease type, disease duration, severity of lesions, age, education level and intelligence) employed by the different researchers and the level of difficulty of the naming tests used in the assessment of MS subjects may have contributed to the discrepant findings relating to naming abilities in MS reported in the literature. Findings of a milder naming impairment in the relapsing-remitting (RR) MS group have led some researchers to suggest that naming abilities may reflect the course of the disease as the prevalence of dysnomia is much higher among chronically progressive (CP) MS subjects (Beatty et al., 1989). The finding of naming deficits in the MS subjects of the present study may have been attributed to a subgroup of language impaired individuals possibly composed of individuals with a CP disease course as suggested in the literature. Indeed, Lethlean and Murdoch (1994b) reported that their subjects with a chronically progressive disease course achieved significantly lower naming scores on the BNT than subjects with a relapsing-remitting disease course.

Naming difficulties, such as those experienced by some of our MS subjects, may be attributed to a semantic access problem or a semantic disorganization problem (LeDorze and Nespoulous, 1989). It has been proposed that there are several types of anomia resulting from different underlying deficits disrupting different processes involved in lexical access and production (LeDorze and Nespoulous, 1989). Lethlean and Murdoch (1994a) examined the types of naming errors produced by subjects with MS and concluded that naming errors in MS may result from disruption at the levels of the perceptual and the semantic system.

Dysfunction in the comprehension of logico-grammatical constructions, apparent in the MS subjects included in our expanded study, is consistent with FitzGerald et al.'s (1987) MS group's performance on the

WST. It is suggested, however, that while statistically the MS subjects, as a group ($M = 46.05$), performed significantly differently from the control group ($M = 49.10$), the clinical meaningfulness of this difference is questionable. A difference of just over three points out of a total score of 50 is not necessarily indicative of comprehension deficits.

Although conceptual and abstract reasoning difficulties have been reported in neuropsychological research studies considering the cognitive abilities of people with MS (e.g. Anzola et al., 1990), previous studies have failed to consider verbal reasoning and associated high level language abilities in their assessments. It is suggested that the significant difficulties on subtests of TWT, experienced by some of our MS subjects, may reflect impaired verbal conceptual reasoning abilities (Jorgensen et al., 1981) or mental inflexibility (Blonder et al., 1989). The MS group attained significantly lower scores when compared to the control group on TWT tasks A, C, E and F, which required the subjects to make associations, explain absurdities and define words. Their inadequate explanations in response to TWT tasks demonstrated impaired verbal reasoning skills and an inability to express critical semantic attributes of their lexicon (Jorgensen et al., 1981). For example, in the Associations task, some MS subjects were able to select a word from a group of four which did not belong to the category, but had difficulty verbalizing the reason behind why the selected item did not belong to the category. Other subjects selected the incorrect word and provided an inadequate reason for why the item was selected. In one test item, subject 6 first had to comprehend and perceptualize the items 'wheel', 'rectangle', 'circle' and 'square'. She then had to recognize that the category was names of shapes and not objects representing these shapes. However, she responded incorrectly with 'rectangle' and gave the reason 'the others are round'. Blonder et al. (1989) have suggested that the failure to provide a second meaning for a target word through categorization and reclassification, as identified in the MS group's performance on task F of TWT, reflects mental inflexibility in language processing.

According to Wiig and Secord (1985), low scores achieved on all the TLC subtests, as identified in our MS group, can be considered to reflect difficulties in divergent language production, impaired planning and problem-solving, and cognitive-linguistic inflexibility. The MS subjects, as a group, had difficulty understanding ambiguous sentences in the TLC and determining two meanings for each sentence when compared to the control subjects. Some MS cases identified a single interpretation of the sentence, however, even with prompting, then failed to evaluate, plan and process a second meaning. Other MS subjects simply gave one response and made no attempt to formulate another response, whereas some individuals provided two answers but with similar meaning. For example, subject 5's two interpretations of the lexically ambiguous sentence 'and you believe Mary wanted to run as well as me' were that Mary 'wanted to be in a race' or 'wanted to compete in one she couldn't go in'.

The MS subjects included in our expanded study also performed more poorly on the Making Inferences subtest of the TLC when compared to the control group, which appeared to reflect inactive processing and an inability to generate hypotheses (Wiig and Secord, 1985). The MS subjects, as a group, had difficulty processing two statements relating a story in order to complete a carrier phrase which required the subject to select, from four multiple-choice options, which sentence best explained what could have occurred in the event. For example, in item 9 of the Making Inferences subtest the subjects were given the statements 'On his way to work, Mr. Brown was happy to see a pancake house ahead. He walked out of the donut shop with a cup of coffee and a donut' and were required to complete the carrier phrase 'Mr. Brown went to the donut shop because' by selecting from four options '(a) a pancake house does not serve breakfast, (b) he did not have time for a complete breakfast, (c) he couldn't get enough to eat at a pancake house and (d) the pancake house had gone out of business'. Some MS subjects were found to select two inappropriate inferences, whereas other subjects were able to identify one plausible inference but failed to select a second appropriate response.

Although the MS subjects and the control group investigated in our expanded study attained similar scores on the gross measure of sentence construction incorporated in the NCCEA, the control subjects performed significantly better than the MS subjects on a more sensitive measure of sentence construction, namely the Recreating Sentences subtest of the TLC. Recreating sentences in the TLC requires the use of three lexical units which must be incorporated in a response appropriate to a common situation. Some of the MS subjects had difficulty with this task and produced sentences that were awkward, incomplete, and/or semantically, pragmatically and syntactically inconsistent. For example, for the recreation of a sentence using the words 'difficult', 'nonetheless' and 'now' in the context of moving house, subject 1 produced the sentence 'Although it was difficult to move now nonetheless it was difficult to do so.' Other subjects had significantly more difficulty using all three words provided when compared with controls.

Results of previous studies have also identified sentence construction difficulties in the MS population (FitzGerald et al., 1987). According to Bock (1982), planning for language production, as required by the

Recreating Sentences subtest of the TLC, requires conceptual integration and synthesis of semantic, syntactic, pragmatic and phonological information. It is suggested that the poor performance of the MS group on the Recreating Sentences subtest may be indicative of the subjects' use of inefficient strategies employed to complete the task, perhaps reflecting cognitive deficits (e.g. short-term memory loss or impaired problem-solving), and/or the subjects' difficulties in accessing, integrating and monitoring linguistic information.

The performance of our MS group on the Metaphor subtest of the TLC was not as competent when compared to the performance of a control group on the same task. The MS subjects made more errors than the control subjects when explaining the meanings of metaphorical expressions. For example, when subject 34 was asked to interpret the metaphor 'She is easily crushed,' he responded 'She is easy to talk into anything.' It is suggested that the MS group's performance on this task reflected poor verbal explanation abilities because performance improved when the MS subjects were required to match metaphoric expressions with the same underlying meaning. Indeed, Wiig and Secord (1985) have suggested that difficulty interpreting metaphoric expressions reflects a reduced ability to problem solve and utilize contextual cues to determine meanings of non-literal language.

The relatively intact reading and writing abilities demonstrated by the MS subjects included in our expanded study are consistent with other group study findings reported in the literature. Other researchers, however, have reported reading and writing deficits in both MS case studies (e.g. Friedman et al., 1983; Day et al., 1987) and group MS studies (Jambor, 1969). Further conclusions concerning reading and writing functions in MS are limited considering that only a subgroup of the MS subjects examined were able to carry out the reading and writing subtests of the NCCEA because of their sensory and motor impairments. In addition, the NCCEA only assessed basic functional reading and writing skills.

In summary, the MS subjects included in our expanded study were found to present with relatively intact performance on a gross measure of aphasia, namely the NCCEA, with the exception of the Word Fluency and Sentence Repetition NCCEA subtests. The use of more sensitive high-level language measures, however, revealed that the MS subjects, as a group, presented with impaired naming and had significant difficulties completing verbal reasoning and linguistic problem-solving tasks. Considering that individual MS subjects in the present study performed within normal limits on the naming tasks, it is suggested that the group results indicating the presence of language problems in MS may reflect the impaired performance of a subgroup of linguistically impaired MS subjects such as suggested by Blackwood et al. (1991). In the literature, the presence of cognitive deficits in individuals with MS has been correlated with disease variables such as disease course, disease duration, degree of disability and so on. It is possible that linguistic deficits in MS may also be related to the presence of particular disease variables. The relationship between MS disease variables, such as disease course, and the MS subjects' performance on naming and high-level language tests will be considered in Chapters 8 and 9.

The results of our study did not identify MS subjects with a typical aphasic syndrome as has been documented in case studies in the literature (e.g. Achiron et al., 1992). The MS subjects, as a group, presented with difficulties in performing complex naming tasks and linguistic assessments relying on the interdependence of language and cognitive functions. Indeed, the influence of cognitive deficits is important to consider as individuals with MS have been reported to present with subcortical dementia (Rao, 1986; Tolosa and Alvarez, 1992), intentional dementia (Nadeau, 1991) or a combination of cortical and subcortical dementia (Beatty et al., 1989).

The linguistic deficits identified in our MS group seem to be representative of a more diffuse brain impairment associated with white matter demyelination in MS. The finding of language difficulties in subjects with MS lends support to the suggestion that the integrity of white matter pathways is necessary in order for normal language processing to take place. Indeed, further discussion of high-level language deficits in relation to models with subcortical white matter pathway involvement in language processing is presented in Chapter 8.

Clinical implications

Awareness of the presence of mild language deficits in individuals with MS is important for speech/language pathologists involved in the rehabilitation of those people who have this disease. The findings of our study are indicative of the need for researchers and clinicians to use more sensitive language assessments than those used in previously reported studies to accurately quantify and describe the linguistic abilities of individuals with MS. The presence of disturbed language abilities in MS has important implications for rehabilitation and management of patients with MS in that language disorders may have a considerable negative impact on an individual's daily life. It is essential, therefore, that clinicians take into account when planning their management of clients with MS the impact of possible language impairments on such activities as work, self-care, interpersonal relationships and other aspects of social life beyond the physical disability associated with MS. Further recogni-

tion of those people with MS who present with high-level language difficulties will then enable clinicians to develop and make available rehabilitation strategies aimed at maximizing language skills.

Chapter 8
High-level language, naming and discourse abilities in multiple sclerosis

BRUCE E MURDOCH AND JENNIFER B LETHLEAN

Introduction

Controversy surrounds the existence of language problems in individuals with multiple sclerosis (MS). Although some single case studies of acute aphasia (Olmos-Lau et al., 1977; Friedman et al., 1983; Day et al., 1987) as well as some group studies (FitzGerald et al., 1987; Blackwood et al., 1991; Lethlean and Murdoch, 1993) have provided evidence in support of the presence of language deficits in MS, other reports have indicated that language disorders rarely occur in this disease (Farmakides and Boone, 1960; Herderschee et al., 1987; Anzola et al., 1990; Jennekens-Schinkel, Lanser et al., 1990; Rao et al., 1991). In the previous chapter of this book (see Chapter 7), however, it was established that although individuals with MS perform largely within normal limits on gross measures of language (e.g. the Neurosensory Centre Comprehensive Examination for Aphasia, Spreen and Benton, 1969), as a group, they present with high-level language deficits on the Test of Language Competence (TLC) (Wiig and Secord, 1985) and The Word Test (TWT) (Jorgensen et al., 1981). More specifically, the people with MS were reported to experience difficulties on tasks which required problem-solving, planning, decision-making and abstract reasoning, thereby also confirming reports in the literature of the presence of subtle cognitive deficits in MS (Rao, 1986; Rao et al., 1991).

Lethlean and Murdoch (1993) proposed that a major reason for the controversial findings concerning language problems in MS is a methodological problem of subject selection where subjects included in the reported studies present with different disease variables. As described in Chapter 1, individuals with MS are commonly separated into two clinical groups, namely those with a relapsing-remitting (RR) disease course and those with a chronically progressive (CP) disease course (Miller et al., 1991), and some researchers have suggested that cognitive and associated language difficulties are closely linked to disease course (Feinstein et al., 1992). Cognitive difficulties have been reported to be more prevalent in individuals with a CP course of MS (Heaton et al., 1985; Jennekens-Schinkel, Lanser et al., 1990; Ron and Feinstein, 1992) and less severe (Beatty, Goodkin et al., 1989; Anzola et al., 1990) or rarely experienced in the RR form of the disease (Heaton et al., 1985; Feinstein et al., 1992). It is possible that language function may also be related to disease course as the linguistically impaired MS individuals identified by Blackwood et al. (1991) and Lethlean and Murdoch (1993) consisted of subjects with a CP disease course. It is possible that previously reported group studies may have masked the presence of MS individuals with normal language function and failed to identify those subjects with more severe language deficits than the group results indicated.

The neuroanatomical basis of cognitive dysfunction in the MS population has been discussed at length in the literature. There have been high correlations between cognitive impairment and brain pathology determined on magnetic resonance imaging (MRI) (e.g. Rao, Leo et al., 1989; Huber et al., 1992), computerized tomography (CT) (e.g. Rao et al., 1985; Rabins et al., 1986) and positron emission tomography (PET) (e.g. Brooks et al., 1984; Pozzilli, Bastianello et al., 1991) in cases of MS. Neuropsychological deficits in individuals with MS have been associated with demyelination of white matter pathways travelling from the prefrontal cortex (Mendez and Frey, 1992). Atrophy of the corpus callosum has also been significantly related to cognitive impairment in MS (Huber et al., 1987; Pozzilli, Bastianello et al., 1991; Huber et al., 1992). Indeed, MS plaques are often found in the frontal lobe and lateral periventricular white matter, which may disconnect subcortical structures from the cerebral cortex (Filley et al., 1989). According to White (1990), considering that MS can extensively involve the subcortical and cortical white matter, thereby interrupting connections to the cortex, it is reasonable to propose that MS subjects will present with symptoms of language loss as well as cognitive deficits.

Researchers have reported that language disorders may result from brain damage affecting structures below the level of the cerebral cortex and that white matter pathways connecting subcortical structures, such as the thalamus, basal ganglia and internal capsule, plus those connecting subcortical structures with the cortex, play an important role in language functions (Crosson, 1985; Metter et al., 1988). Subcortical structures have been incorporated into models of language processing (Crosson, 1985; Wallesch and Papagno, 1988) and the cortico-subcortico-cortical loop has been described as being involved in the integration of information (Wallesch and Papagno, 1988) and subcortical modulation of cortical activity (Crosson, 1985; Metter et al., 1988; Wallesch and Papagno, 1988). Given that MS white matter lesions correlate with cognitive deficits and are well placed to disconnect the subcortical and cortical structures, it is possible that demyelination and associated disconnection of the cortico-subcortico-cortical loop may result in high-level language dysfunction.

High-level language abilities in multiple sclerosis: effect of disease course

The most extensive study of the high-level language abilities of persons with MS conducted to date is that reported by Lethlean and Murdoch (1997). They described the high-level language abilities in chronic MS using a larger sample of MS subjects than that examined by Lethlean and Murdoch (1993) and investigated the relationship between the presence of language disorders and disease course. In order to provide further insight into the role of subcortical white matter pathways in language function, Lethlean and Murdoch (1997) also discussed the observed language problems with reference to contemporary models of subcortical participation in language processing. Consequently, this section of the present chapter will focus on providing a synthesis of the findings of Lethlean and Murdoch (1997). The subjects examined by Lethlean and Murdoch (1997) were the same 60 individuals with a diagnosis of definite MS described in Chapter 7. The personal details of the MS subjects including their age, sex, education, age at onset of first MS symptoms, age at diagnosis, duration of disease and medications are shown in Tables 7.2 and 7.3. Sixty non-neurologically impaired individuals matched for age, sex, education level and professional status served as controls.

Each of the MS subjects was classified according to their disease course into either a chronically progressive (CP) or relapsing-remitting (RR) group. Subjects were assigned to the CP group if they had experienced a history of gradual deterioration of physical abilities where symptoms had progressively become worse. Subjects were included in the RR group if they reported a disease course with relapses and remissions where symptoms had occurred for a short period of time and then improved. Thirty-two subjects (53%) were classified as having a CP disease course (mean age 52 ± 12 years, range 28–76 years; mean level of education 12 ± 2 years, range 6–17 years) and 28 subjects (47%) were included in the RR group (mean age 45 ± 11 years, range 26–66 years; mean level of education 12 ± 2 years, range 10–16 years). For the CP group, the mean duration of the disease since the onset of MS was 19 ±

12 years, ranging from 1 to 53 years, and for the RR group was 12 ± 10 years, ranging from 1 to 41 years. The average age at which first symptoms occurred in the CP group was 33 ± 13 years, ranging from 16 to 64 years, and in the RR group was 33 ± 9 years ranging from 20 to 55 years. The average age at diagnosis for the CP subjects was 39 ± 13 years ranging from 20 to 65 years, and for the RR subjects was 37 ± 10 years, ranging from 20 to 56 years.

The test battery administered by Lethlean and Murdoch (1997) included the Test of Language Competence (TLC) (Wiig and Secord, 1985) and The Word Test (TWT) (Jorgensen et al., 1981). Each subject completed the assessments over two sessions and the maximum length of a testing session was one and a half hours. The MS subjects with a RR course of the disease were assessed during a period of disease remission. Testing was discontinued and completed in a subsequent session if the subject became fatigued and all language tests were carried out under standard conditions in constant and quiet surroundings.

The TLC was designed to identify young people (aged nine and above), and adults with language disabilities. The test incorporates assessments of semantics, syntax, and pragmatics using formats that probe divergent production, cognitive-linguistic flexibility and planning for production. Tasks included require problem-solving, planning and decision-making and/or alternative solutions or responses to the same linguistic input. The subtests of the TLC require interpretation of ambiguous sentences, making inferences, recreating sentences, and interpretation of figurative language. It was considered that these tasks reflect high-level language abilities because they entail the use of varied areas of language and extensive cognitive processing. Five subjects were unable to complete subtest 2 (Making Inferences) and one subject was unable to complete subtest 4 (Understanding Metaphoric Expressions) because of their visual problems and resulting reading difficulties. All subjects were presented with both visual and auditory input for all subtests. For example, in subtest 1 (Understanding Ambiguous Sentences) the sentences were presented in written form and then read out by the examiner. A sentence was then repeated several times if required by the subject.

Although TWT was developed for school-aged children, it was included in the test battery as it provides an indication of subjects' abilities to recognize and express the critical semantic attributes of their lexicon through the processes of categorizing, defining, verbal reasoning and choosing appropriate words. Indeed, Jorgensen et al. (1981) suggested that TWT can determine areas of verbal strengths and weaknesses in an aphasic adult's performance, especially those whose overall function is within the performance range of the assessment. All subjects in the study reported by Lethlean and Murdoch (1997) were able to complete the TWT.

The results of the high-level language tests administered by Lethlean and Murdoch (1997) indicated that, as a group, the subjects with MS presented with difficulties understanding ambiguous sentences and metaphoric expressions, making inferences, and recreating sentences, and exhibited relatively poor performance on voluntary and semantic tasks compared to the controls. Further, Lethlean and Murdoch (1997) reported that individuals with either a CP or RR disease course both had significant high-level language problems. In particular, the division of the MS subjects into groups according to disease course, revealed that individuals with both a CP and a RR course experienced significantly more difficulties than the control group when interpreting ambiguities and metaphors, recreating sentences and forming inferences. Irrespective of disease course, the MS subjects also performed more poorly than the controls on the vocabulary and semantic tasks of TWT including making associations, explaining absurdities, identifying antonyms, and defining words. The occurrence of high-level language difficulties in MS was not specifically determined by disease course as has been previously suggested by some authors (Feinstein et al., 1992). The findings of Lethlean and Murdoch's (1997) investigation did, however, indicate that individuals with a CP disease course may present with more severe high-level language difficulties when compared to a RR group. Further examination of the results revealed that only the CP group performed more poorly than the control group on the Synonym task of TWT. Overall, the CP group was more severely impaired on the Recreating Sentences and Understanding Ambiguous Sentences subtests of the TLC and on the Associations, Synonyms and Multiple Definition tasks of TWT.

Although the differences between the performance of the CP and RR MS subjects and the control group on subtests of TWT were statistically significant, the magnitude of the differences and the clinical meaningfulness of some of the observed differences were questioned by Lethlean and Murdoch (1997). For example, differences in the means of the subjects' identification of synonyms and antonyms in all three groups were less than two points out of a ceiling score of 16 and 14, respectively. It was proposed by Lethlean and Murdoch (1997) that the TLC revealed more clinically relevant high-level language deficits in their CP and RR MS groups and, therefore, consideration of the MS subjects' performances on the TLC will form the basis of the following theoretical discussion.

According to Bernstein (1987), the use of non-literal language such as ambiguity, metaphorical expressions and so on, acts to add a depth and richness to language and allows subtle indirect communication of information. The way in which people process figurative language is a complex procedure, which has been discussed and debated at length in the literature (Baldwin et al., 1982; Bernstein, 1987; Frazier and Rayner, 1987; Simpson and Krueger, 1991), and results so far have been inconclusive.

Lethlean and Murdoch (1997) noted that both the RR and the CP MS subjects had difficulty identifying two meanings for ambiguous sentences in the TLC. Illustrative examples of the test items include 'And then the man wiped the glasses carefully' (lexical ambiguity); 'Bob did not blame the girl as much as her mother' (surface structure ambiguity); and 'I have always known that flying planes can be dangerous' (deep structure ambiguity). For each of these items, the subjects were required to produce two possible meanings for the sentences without contextual cues. For example, the sentence 'And then the man wiped the glasses carefully' is ambiguous because there is no contextual information which suggests whether or not the lexically ambiguous word 'glasses' refers to 'reading glasses' or 'drinking glasses'. Some of the MS subjects were able to identify one correct meaning but, even with prompting, failed to evaluate, plan and process a second interpretation of the sentence. Other MS subjects provided two responses but with similar meanings.

Researchers have attempted to explain the normal process of individuals' understanding of lexically ambiguous language (Simpson, 1984; Burgess and Simpson, 1988). Indeed, there is considerable debate in the literature as to whether or not the comprehension of ambiguity is interactive (i.e. dependent on context) or modular. A review completed by Simpson (1984) has outlined the three major models for ambiguous processing. The first model is the context dependent or selective access model, which is an interactive model proposing that the meanings of ambiguous words are stimulated by the context of the sentence in which they occur (Glucksberg et al., 1986). In this context dependent model only the contextually appropriate meaning of the ambiguous word is accessed (Simpson, 1981; Simpson et al., 1989). Another model is the single access model which suggests that the meanings of an ambiguous word are retrieved serially according to their frequency (Hogaboam and Perfetti, 1975). That is, the most frequent meaning is accessed first and if the meaning is appropriate in context the search is discontinued. If, however, the retrieved meaning is not appropriate in context the search continues to another meaning and so on. In the absence of contextual information the most frequent meaning is activated first.

The modular based multiple access model for ambiguous processing proposed by Onifer and Swinney (1981), however, seems to be the one best applied to the model of language processing, outlined by Wallesch and Papagno (1988), which incorporates cortical and subcortical structures and their connections. In turn, Lethlean and Murdoch (1997) suggested that Wallesch and Papagno's (1988) model helped to explain the poor performance by their MS subjects on the understanding ambiguous sentences task of the TLC. According to Onifer and Swinney's (1981) model of ambiguous processing, all meanings are simultaneously activated upon presentation of an ambiguous word. Once the meanings of the word have been accessed the context influences the selection of the appropriate meaning.

In Wallesch and Papagno's (1988) model of language processing, parallel neuroanatomical modules provide alternatives (e.g. different meanings for an ambiguous sentence) which are transmitted to the thalamus via the globus pallidus. Only one response, however, is released by the thalamus to be produced by the cortex. The parallel modules originating in the cortex form cortico-striato-pallido-thalamo-cortical loops, which enable the production of alternative interpretations of ambiguous items. Lethlean and Murdoch (1997) proposed that interruptions to the cortico-subcortical pathways within a modular system may have resulted in the MS subjects' failure to provide alternative meanings for the ambiguous sentences. In some of their MS cases, it was suggested that only some of the modular pathways were interrupted so that, while a single module completed the circuit and the cortex produced one meaning of the ambiguous sentence, a second meaning was not generated or accessed. For example, subject 8's two similar interpretations of the lexically ambiguous sentence 'I knew that glare really bothered Jane' were 'the glare from the sun' or 'the glare from the light reflecting off the glass'.

The interpretation of syntactically ambiguous sentences has been found to be heavily influenced by the prosodic patterns used by the speaker (Beach, 1991). The subtest of the TLC requiring the interpretation of syntactically ambiguous sentences, however, did not provide the intonation or phrasing cues for the subjects examined by Lethlean and Murdoch (1997). Indeed, both their CP and RR MS subjects had difficulty identifying two meanings for ambiguous sentences with deep and surface structure ambiguities. For example, subject 16 had difficulty providing two meanings for the sentence, 'The man was sure that the duck was ready to eat.' She gave two interpretations with similar meanings, namely, 'It was cooked' and 'It'd been plucked'. In the absence of prosodic information, it is possible that the syntactically ambiguous sentences are processed in a modular way, similar to lexically ambiguous sentences, where the two potential meanings are determined based on the information given by the cortex and integrated and organized by the subcortical structures according to Wallesch and Papagno's (1988) model of language processing. It is recognized, however, that within each module it is likely that different processes will be carried out for lexical versus syntactic ambiguities.

The CP and the RR MS subjects tested by Lethlean and Murdoch (1997) experienced more difficulty than control subjects when explaining metaphorical expressions in the TLC. For example, when subject 48 was asked to interpret the metaphor 'There is rough sailing ahead for us' in the situation 'Two students moving into a new town', she responded: 'There is a rough area ahead for them.' According to Bernstein (1987), the term metaphor means to carry over meaning, and the comprehension of a metaphor requires the individual to convey aspects of one object over to another object so that it is spoken of as the first object. Gentner (1983) described three types of metaphors namely, attribute, relational, and double metaphors. The metaphorical expressions in the TLC consist of relational metaphors in which the topic and vehicle share a relationship. In the example 'There is rough sailing ahead for us', the relationship between the topic 'moving to a new town' and the vehicle 'going in a sailing boat in rough weather' is that both express the notion of 'the future' and of 'difficulties'. Lethlean and Murdoch (1997) suggested that their MS subjects' difficulty in the figurative language tasks may not necessarily reflect an inability to understand these metaphorical relationships but rather that their difficulty is a reflection of poor verbal explanation abilities. Indeed, the subjects' performances improved when they were required to match metaphorical expressions such as 'There is rough sailing ahead for us' with similar underlying meanings from a choice of four items: one a correct match (e.g. 'We will be facing a hard road'), and three distracters representing an opposite metaphor (e.g. 'The rough times are behind us now'), a literal interpretation (e.g. 'The waves are going to make it hard to sail'), and a non-related metaphor (e.g. 'It took the wind out of our sails'). Children have also been found to perform better on a multiple choice task of understanding metaphors than verbally explaining metaphors (Bernstein, 1987).

Bernstein (1987) has suggested that the metaphorical expressions in the TLC are more idiomatic in nature. While an idiomatic phrase can be interpreted literally, when it is used in a particular context it may express a non-literal idea or a concept (Bernstein, 1987). Van Lancker and Canter (1981) have suggested that idioms are processed as one unit which is perceived and expressed differently from the literal interpretation of the same phrase. Indeed, an example in the TLC such as 'It's still up in the air' may be viewed as an unconscious idiom which is routinely used in language. It has been reported that the comprehension of idioms relates highly to an individual's exposure to them, the linguistic context in which the idiom is presented, and also the way in which comprehension of idioms is assessed (Bernstein, 1987). Lethlean and Murdoch (1977) drew attention to the fact that the TLC is an American-based test, leading them to suggest that the reason their Australian control and MS subjects both had difficulty on some items of the Understanding Metaphorical Expressions subtest was that they had not been exposed to some of the American expressions. For example, some subjects made no attempt to interpret the expression 'He is high man on the totem pole' because they had never heard the expression before.

There is currently debate in the literature as to whether or not a non-literal interpretation of a metaphor is accessed directly in context or whether it is preceded by a literal interpretation (Winner, 1988). Glucksberg (1989) has suggested that literal and figurative expressions have similar recognition problems and depend equally on contextual information and that a non-literal interpretation does not depend on the previously accessed literal meaning. Indeed, literal comprehension has been found to be unrelated to the understanding of metaphors in head injured (Dennis and Barnes, 1990) and language learning disabled adolescents (Jones and Stone, 1989). Dennis and Barnes (1990) found that the metaphors were not converted to literal language before being understood by the closed head injury group. In relation to Wallesch and Papagno's (1988) model, Lethlean and Murdoch (1997) speculated that subjects interpreting metaphors would possibly access both the literal and non-literal interpretations simultaneously in the form of different modules travelling via cortico-striato-pallido-thalamo-cortical pathways. The contextual information also supplied by the cortex to the integrating and gating subcortical structures would enable selection of the metaphorical meaning in the module appropriate for the situation.

Lethlean and Murdoch (1997) suggested that organizational linguistic difficulties were reflected in their CP and RR MS group's signif-icantly poor performance on the Recreating Sentences subtest of the TLC. Some of their MS subjects had difficulty integrating and organizing three words which had to be incorporated into a sentence in a given context. For example, each subject had to formulate a sentence with the words 'difficult' 'nonetheless' and 'now' in the context of 'moving house'. A picture of the scenario 'moving house' was provided for the subjects with the words printed above the picture. In addition, the context and the words were read aloud by the examiner. Certain MS subjects were found to have difficulty including all three words in the construction of their sentences and so produced an intact sentence with one or two of the words. For example, subject 16 constructed the sentence 'It was difficult job packing up nonetheless it will be for the better.' Other subjects attempted to include all three words but produced sentences which were awkward, incomplete and/or semantically, pragmatically and syntactically inconsistent. For example, subject 13 produced the non-sentence 'Nonetheless the last furniture had to go now being difficult.' The findings of sentence construction difficulties in MS subjects by Lethlean and Murdoch (1997) support previous findings (e.g. FitzGerald et al., 1987). Indeed, Bock (1982) has suggested that recreating sentences demands conceptual integration and synthesis of semantic, pragmatic and syntactic variables. Lethlean and Murdoch (1997) proposed that their MS subjects' poor performance on the recreating sentence items of the TLC may reflect inefficient strategies used to complete the task (with a possible cognitive origin) and/or difficulties in integrating and monitoring linguistic information.

Pathology of the neostriatum has been found to disturb syntactic organization of language production and linguistic processing in Huntington's disease (Illes, 1989). Gordon (1985) suggested that the linguistic deficits in Huntington's disease may result from disconnection of afferents from the superior temporal gyrus to the head of the caudate nucleus. One of the roles of the basal ganglia in language processing outlined in Wallesch and Papagno's (1988) model is one of integrating and monitoring linguistic information. It is suggested that with the potential disconnection of the cortical structures from subcortical input, due to demyelination of subcortical white matter pathways in MS, the cortex would have difficulty organizing and integrating the three words into a syntactically, semantically and pragmatically appropriate sentence. Lethlean and Murdoch (1997) speculated that the compromised performance of their MS subjects on the sentence construction task of the TLC, which required the application of internalized morphologic and syntactic rules (Wiig and Semel, 1974), may have been related to poor intentional self monitoring abilities. Indeed, a goal-directed intentional role of the deep subcortical nuclei has been proposed by Wallesch (1985) where the will of an individual must be integrated when formulating language.

The CP and RR MS subjects studied by Lethlean and Murdoch (1997) also performed significantly below the control group on the TLC subtest of Making Inferences. The subjects were required to read two statements relating a story and then complete the story by choosing from four inferences which best explained what could have happened. The statements and inferential choices were read out by the examiner to ensure that the items were read accurately. According to Wiig and Secord (1985), reduced scores on this inferential subtest of the TLC, as demonstrated by Lethlean and Murdoch's (1997) MS group, represent inactive processing and an inability to generate hypotheses.

Dennis and Barnes (1990), on the basis of their assessment of a closed head injury group, found that the ability of a subject to make inferences was highly predictable from a knowledge of the individual's working memory and that poor inferencing skills may have significant implications for discourse. Dennis and Barnes (1990) suggested that if an individual has a poor working memory, as may occur in MS (e.g. Minden et al., 1990) especially in accessing information from primary memory (Rao, St Aubin-Faubert et al., 1989), comprehension of text and situation will continually be overtaxed because even situations which have been already presented must be constantly understood anew. For example, by the time the MS subjects tested by Lethlean and Murdoch (1997) reached the choices of inferences provided in the TLC they may have been unable to remember the situation from which they were making inferences. Unfortunately, the results of a comprehensive neuropsychological evaluation of cognitive functions (including memory) of the MS subjects included in their study were not available to Lethlean and Murdoch (1997).

The MS subjects examined by Lethlean and Murdoch (1997) presented with difficulties on linguistic subtests relying on the inter-dependence of language and cognitive functions (Wiig and Secord, 1985). However, limited data regarding the MS individuals' cognitive abilities and the possibility of a concomitant dementia in MS (e.g. Tolosa and Alvarez, 1992), restrict the conclusions which can be made concerning the basis of their high-level language deficits. Lethlean and Murdoch (1997) recommend that further investigation of high-level language abilities in MS be carried out incorporating both neuropsycho-logical and language assessments.

Other MS disease variables such as severity of disability, disease duration, drug regimens, and number, site and extent of white matter lesions, not examined by Lethlean and Murdoch (1997), may have also contributed to the presence of linguistic difficulties in their MS group. Examination of their MS subjects' results on the TLC and TWT revealed a subgroup of linguistically impaired MS subjects. Indeed, an overall measure of MS severity (e.g. the Expanded Disability Status Scale, Kurtze, 1983b) may have characterized the language disordered MS subgroup better than disease course; however, further discussion of this suggestion was considered by Lethlean and Murdoch (1997) to be beyond the scope of their paper as quantitative neurological assess-ments of MS severity were not carried out. Disease duration has been reported as a variable which may contribute to the diverse performance of MS individuals on cognitive and associated language tasks (e.g. Mendozzi et al., 1993). Various medications used in the treatment of MS symptoms (e.g. benzodiazepines, tricyclic antidepressants and antiepileptics) have been found to affect speech, word retrieval, and higher cognitive processing (Hodgson, 1993). Therefore, evaluation of the potential effects of specific medications on MS subjects' performance on language tasks may be a worthwhile topic for future investigations. There have been a number of studies which have documented significant correlations between the site and extent of MS white matter lesions apparent on neuroradiological examination and MS subjects' performance on neuropsychological assessments (e.g. Swirsky-Sacchetti et al., 1992). It is possible that the language deficits identified in the present MS subjects may relate to site and number of focal areas of demyelination in the CNS. Definitive answers, however, can only be arrived at following further studies correlating quantitative measures of lesion load on MRI and scores on language tasks. Indeed, further research is required to determine the characteristics of the identified language impaired MS subgroup including comprehensive neurological, neuroradiological and neuropsychological assessments in relation to language performance.

Lethlean and Murdoch (1997) concluded that the high-level language dysfunction identified in their MS groups appears to be representative of a more diffuse brain impairment associated with white matter demyelination in MS. Although the diffuse and variable involvement of the cerebral white matter tracts in MS (Rao et al., 1985) makes it difficult to provide precise statements concerning the anatomical substrate that influences high-level language processing in this disease, it would appear that Wallesch and Papagno's (1988) model of language processing is useful for explaining, in part, the high-level language dysfunction in MS observed by Lethlean and Murdoch (1997). Certainly, the findings of Lethlean and Murdoch (1997) support the suggestion that individuals with interruptions in the subcortical white matter pathways, such as occur in MS, may experience high-level language problems.

Naming abilities in multiple sclerosis

The presence of impaired naming abilities in persons with MS is somewhat controversial. Although some authors (Heaton et al., 1985; Caine et al., 1986; Beatty et al., 1988; Beatty, Goodkin et al., 1989; Beatty and Monson, 1989; Blackwood et al., 1991; Pozzilli, Bastianello et al., 1991; Lethlean and Murdoch, 1993, 1994a, b) have identified naming impairments in individuals with MS, others have reported intact naming abilities in this population (Herderschee et al., 1987; Callanan et al., 1989; Ron et al., 1991). Factors such as disease course, disease duration, age, education level, site of lesion, degree of neurological impairment and physical disability, and the residential status (e.g. residing at home or in hospital) of the MS subjects at the time of assessment have been implicated as subject variables that might contribute to the varied research findings (Lethlean and Murdoch 1994b).

Errors on picture naming tests produced by neurologically impaired groups have been attributed to a breakdown in any or some combination of perceptual, semantic, and lexical components of naming a picture (LaBarge et al., 1992). Researchers have suggested that the process of accurate picture naming requires efficient perceptual, semantic and lexical cognitive analyses (Snodgrass, 1984). According to LaBarge et al. (1992), in order to name pictures, subjects are required to perceptually analyse the visual features of the picture. They must then determine the underlying conceptual representation of the picture and then proceed to access the appropriate name from the lexicon.

Individuals with primarily subcortical grey matter disease, interrupting normal subcortical function (e.g. Parkinson's disease and supranuclear palsy), have been found to present with paraphasic errors on confrontation naming tasks (Obler, 1983). Obler (1983) suggested that where naming impairment is present in individuals with subcortical dementia, the naming errors may be attributed, in part, to inattention. Considering that MS individuals have been found to present with subcortical dementia (Tolosa and Alvarez, 1992), it is proposed that MS subjects with white matter interruption to normal subcortical function may present with similar 'inattention' naming errors. Other researchers, however, have suggested that the profile of dementia associated with MS consists of neuropsychological deficits found in both cortical and subcortical dementia (Beatty et al., 1990). It is possible that in the absence of normal subcortical influences on the cortex, the naming errors produced by the MS group may also reflect similar errors resulting from cortical dysfunction.

The most comprehensive studies of the naming abilities of persons with MS completed to date are those reported by Lethlean and Murdoch (1994a, b). In one of these studies, the authors examined the effects of variables such as disease course, disease duration, age, and education level on naming abilities in MS (Lethlean and Murdoch, 1994b), while in the other study they examined the nature of naming errors produced by an MS group. In both studies the subjects were the same 60 individuals with MS as described in the investigations of language abilities reported in Chapter 7 (see Tables 7.2 and 7.3 for full descriptions of their personal and medical details).

The findings of Lethlean and Murdoch (1994b) confirmed the presence of a naming deficit in MS. Further, they reported that MS subjects with either a CP or RR disease course attained significantly lower scores on the Boston Naming Test (BNT) (Kaplan et al., 1983) when compared to a control group. The results also indicated that the CP subjects, as a group, achieved BNT scores significantly below the RR group, suggesting that naming was more severely impaired in the CP group. Although it has been proposed that the contradictory findings regarding naming abilities of MS subjects reported in the literature may be related to various subject selection criteria, the results of Lethlean and Murdoch's (1994b) study failed to indicate that the presence of naming problems was related to disease course. The suggestion that disease course is not a reliable predictor of naming problems in MS (Franklin et al., 1989; Rao et al., 1991; Capra et al., 1992) was, therefore, supported by the results obtained by Lethlean and Murdoch (1994b). In addition their findings failed to determine any relationship between naming scores and subject variables such as age, education and disease duration.

An investigation of the confrontation naming errors produced by individuals with MS in response to the BNT by Lethlean and Murdoch (1994a) demonstrated that MS subjects made relatively more naming errors, particularly in the major category of semantic errors, than matched controls. The MS group was found, however, to exhibit similar patterns of naming errors to the control group across all error types including semantic, no relationship, perceptual, phonological and unrecognized correct categories.

Classification of confrontation naming errors has been utilized in the literature to explore the basis of the naming impairment in a number of neurologically impaired groups including individuals with Alzheimer's disease (Smith et al., 1989), aphasia following cerebrovascular accidents (Kohn and Goodglass, 1985), closed head injury (Jordan et al., 1990), and posterior fossa tumour (Hudson-Tennent and Murdoch, 1993). Naming difficulties identified in adult brain damaged individuals have been attributed to a lexical 'access' problem (LeDorze and Nespoulous, 1989), a semantic 'disorganization' problem (Smith et al., 1989; LaBarge et al., 1992), or a 'perceptual' deficit (Kirshner et al., 1984). Indeed, the naming errors produced by the MS group examined by Lethlean and Murdoch (1994a) may have resulted from different underlying deficits disrupting different processes involved in lexical access and production, semantic organization, and visual perception.

Based on the findings of Lethlean and Murdoch (1994a), it is suggested that the presence of a semantically based deficit is the most parsimonious explanation for the presence of a significantly greater frequency of semantic error types produced by the MS group when compared to the control group. Lethlean and Murdoch (1994a) proposed that the types of errors produced by their MS group support

Beatty and Monson's (1989) suggestion of impaired 'access' to semantic memory resulting from inefficient patterns of semantic memory search (Caine et al., 1986; Beatty et al., 1989). Indeed, Beatty and Monson (1990) have suggested that naming dysfunction in MS reflects an inability to retrieve the appropriate word from the lexicon, rather than a breakdown of semantic knowledge as has been identified in Alzheimer's disease (Smith et al., 1989).

Naming dysfunction in neurologically impaired groups has been attributed to deterioration in the semantic features of attributes which determine the meaning of a concept within the semantic system (see LaBarge et al., 1992 for discussion regarding perceptual versus semantic deficit hypotheses). This level of breakdown has been reported to result in bizarre, unrelated responses to naming tasks which have been attributed to increasing involvement of core semantic structures (LaBarge et al., 1992). The MS group studied by Lethlean and Murdoch (1994a), however, produced statistically similar numbers of no relationship errors when compared to the control group. The error analysis revealed that very few numbers of wild paraphasias and deviant circumlocutions were produced by the MS subjects suggesting that, as a group, their core semantic structures were relatively intact.

Researchers have suggested that subjects who produce errors which are semantically related to the target word have adequate semantic information concerning the word to retrieve a related incorrect production (LaBarge et al., 1992). The findings reported by Lethlean and Murdoch (1994a) revealed that a majority of the naming errors produced by their MS group, found to be significantly higher in frequency than the control group, reflected semantic errors which were linguistically related to the target word. Semantic paraphasias were the most frequently occurring semantic error type produced by the MS group. Indeed, qualitative examination of the naming errors produced by the MS subjects seems to support the hypothesis of an accessing deficit rather than a semantic organization deficit in MS. Lethlean and Murdoch (1994a) suggested, for example, that the production of the incorrect response 'squirrel' for the target 'beaver' indicates that the subject who provided this semantic paraphasia was able to access sufficient semantic information to retrieve a related but incorrect response. Similarly, another high frequency semantic error which their MS group gave was the production of definitional circumlocutions for the target (e.g. 'hangman's rope' for 'noose'), also suggesting that they had an understanding of the semantic features of the item to be named.

The presence of a lexical 'accessing' deficit in MS rather than a semantic 'organization' deficit contributing to impaired naming is supported by the finding of intact lexical priming in MS subjects (Beatty and Monson, 1990). Poor performance on priming tasks has been attributed to a failure to activate representations in semantic memory (Shimamura et al., 1987). Beatty et al. (1990) found that a group of MS subjects performed within normal limits on priming tasks, even in those cases where subjects presented with naming deficits. It is proposed that the representations of lexical items within the semantic memory store are intact in individuals with MS; however, further study is required to support this suggestion.

Although a semantic accessing deficit appears to be the best explanation for the naming errors produced by the MS subjects examined by Lethlean and Murdoch (1994a), it is suggested that the group study masked the presence of a few MS individuals who produced high frequencies of bizarre, unrelated responses. For example, over 50% of one subject's (subject 23) error responses demonstrated no relationship to the target word. It is possible that those MS subjects who produced many unrelated responses in the naming task may reflect the presence of semantic disorganization, as occurs in the later stages of Alzheimer's disease, possibly associated with diffuse white matter lesions, cognitive deterioration, and the onset of dementia. Indeed, certain cognitive deficits in MS have been associated with periventricular plaques, diffuse cerebral involvement associated with demyelination (Rao et al., 1984; Rao et al., 1985), and atrophy of the corpus callosum (Huber et al., 1987). Hence, it is possible that the resulting dementia in MS may contribute to naming errors similar to the pattern which has been outlined in cortical dementias.

An additional explanation for naming errors in neurologically impaired groups, which may explain some of the errors exhibited by the MS subjects in Lethlean and Murdoch's (1994a) study, is the suggestion of a visual perceptual deficit which causes subjects to provide the name of an item that is similar in appearance to the target (Kirshner et al., 1984). The MS subjects in the study reported by Lethlean and Murdoch (1994a) were found to produce significantly more perceptual errors than the control group although the clinical relevance of the small difference between the means for the two groups is questionable. The authors suggested, however, that some individual MS subjects' errors can be potentially explained by the perceptual hypothesis. For example, subject 15 produced 10 out of a total of 34 error responses (29.4%) which appeared to result from misperceptions of the target word. For example, she perceived the 'whistle' as a 'lawnmower' and responded 'clouds up there' for the target 'volcano' perceiving the smoke from the volcano as clouds in the sky.

Disturbances in visual acuity associated with demyelination of the optic nerve (Rao, 1986) may explain some of the perceptual error responses given by the MS individuals in Lethlean and Murdoch's (1994a) study. Subjects 4, 8, 15, 23, 32 and 59 all reported visual distur-bances which interfered with their ability to read; however, these same subjects reported that they had adequate visual acuity to attempt the naming task. Investigation of the MS subjects' visual form discrimination or any other visual assessment was not completed; therefore, the influ-ence of optic nerve disturbances on the subjects' performance on the naming task was unable to be eliminated. It is interesting to note, however, that Nicholas et al. (1989) have found that some non-brain-damaged adults may find the stimulus pictures in the BNT to be ambiguous or visually confusing. They suggest that when brain-damaged adults misname these items, researchers should be cautious about attributing naming errors to the subjects' brain impairment. Indeed, in the study reported by Lethlean and Murdoch (1994a), many of the control subjects also produced perceptual errors, particularly for the target 'pretzel', which was often perceived by both the control and MS subjects as a 'knot' or a 'worm'. It is also possible that some of the misnamed BNT items occurring in their MS and control groups may be attributed to cultural biases of the picture stimuli reported by some researchers (Worrall and Burtenshaw, 1990). For example, the target 'beaver' on the BNT is likely to be used more frequently in America than in Australia. Indeed, individual subjects in both subject groups were found to produce the relatively high-frequency close contrast coordi-nates 'platypus' and 'wombat' (Australian animals with similar semantic features) rather than the low-frequency target 'beaver'.

Although some MS individuals produced high frequencies of percep-tual errors, the overall number of perceptual errors produced by the MS subjects studied by Lethlean and Murdoch (1994a), as a group, was minimal when compared to the other error types. Within the MS group's error types the perceptual erroneous responses were among the least frequently occurring error type, reflecting a pattern of error types similar to the control group. The perceptual hypothesis, while explaining some of the naming errors in the MS group, failed to account for the signifi-cantly higher frequency of semantic errors when compared to the control group. Studies investigating naming errors in Alzheimer's disease have indicated that the number of misnamings related only visually to the target are less than would be expected if visual-perceptual deficits alone caused the error responses (Schwartz et al., 1979; Bayles and Tomoeda, 1983). In addition, if the visual-perceptual signal was degraded, the errors would be random and only related semantically to the target by chance (Smith et al., 1989). Similarly, Lethlean and Murdoch (1994a) proposed that if a visual-perceptual deficit was the primary basis for the naming errors in their MS group, the MS subjects would have produced relatively larger numbers of perceptual errors and a different pattern of errors in response to the naming task when compared to controls.

The presence of part-whole errors, where a subject mistakenly names a part of the target object, or names the whole that contains the target, has been associated with anomia resulting from frontal damage in brain-injured groups (Kohn and Goodglass, 1985). Indeed, individuals with MS have been found to present with neuropsychological dysfunction associated with demyelination of subcortical white matter pathways emanating from the prefrontal cortex (Mendez and Frey, 1992) potentially disconnecting the frontal hemispheres from subcortical structures. Qualitative examination of the perceptual errors exhibited by the MS group studied by Lethlean and Murdoch (1994a) revealed that many were part-whole perceptual errors (e.g. 'scissors ready to cut something' for 'helicopter' or 'lantern' for 'knocker'), whereas the controls, when they made perceptual errors, tended to produce perceptually related items (e.g. 'snake' for 'pretzel' or 'piece of fruit' for 'acorn'). The semantic feature analysis revealed that the MS group produced more 'functional context' semantic features in responding to a target relative to the controls. For example, MS subjects produced the name of the word 'dog' which is in the functional context of the target 'muzzle'. Lethlean and Murdoch (1994a) suggested that, in some cases, this may have reflected the individual's failure to attend to the target. Indeed, Kohn and Goodglass (1985) have proposed that semantic and perceptual part-whole errors may reflect cognitive attentional deficits where the subjects fail to attend to the correct stimuli. The MS group investigated by Lethlean and Murdoch (1994a), however, produced similar proportions of semantically related part-whole semantic features in response to the target. It is possible that the group study may have masked individuals whose error responses may have reflected inattention associated with disruptions in frontal cortical-subcortical connections.

Obler (1983) proposed that naming errors in subjects with subcortical dementia may reflect their inattention to errors and reduced self monitoring. It was suggested by Lethlean and Murdoch (1994a) that the naming errors produced by the MS subjects in their study may also be related to disrupted subcortical mechanisms and associated attentional and monitoring difficulties. Obler (1983) postulated that inattention causes the subject to access similar semantically close verbal substitutions that most normal subjects will self-correct or inhibit before they are produced. Indeed, this may explain the greater number of semantic errors produced by the MS group compared to the control group in Lethlean and Murdoch's (1994a) study as well as the similar proportions of semantic features occurring in both groups. Considering that subcortical structures have been implicated in the monitoring of language production and that MS tends to interrupt the normal pathways allowing communication between cortical and subcortical structures, compromised naming abilities found in the MS group may be attributed, in part, to poor self-monitoring skills.

Although the lesion sites of their MS subjects were not confirmed by Lethlean and Murdoch (1994a), they suggested that speculative discussion of subcortical mechanisms in relation to language production in MS promoted an explanation worthy of consideration. Indeed, a preverbal semantic monitoring role of the thalamus has been outlined in Crosson's (1985) model of language processing which may, in part, explain the presence of a higher frequency production of semantic errors in the MS group compared to the control group. Crosson (1985) suggested that reciprocal connections between the thalamus and the cortex provide a feedback loop, which enables the temporo-parietal areas of the cortex to monitor the encoding of language before it is produced. Language formulated in the anterior language centre (e.g. the name an MS subject provides for a picture) is transmitted via a cortico-thalamo-cortical pathway to the posterior temporo-parietal language centre which decodes and checks the semantic input. If the name for the item is monitored as inaccurate and requires modification, the semantic information is conveyed via the same pathway back to the anterior cortex to be corrected.

According to Crosson's (1985) model, the basal ganglia perform a motor release function and indirectly modify cortical activity via the thalamus allowing language to be produced. For example, if the name for the target picture is ready for production, having been checked by the temporo-parietal cortex, the temporo-parietal cortex temporarily inhibits the pallidal nuclei of the basal ganglia releasing the thalamus from inhibition. In turn, the thalamus increases its excitatory effect on the anterior cortex permitting the release of the monitored lexical item for motor programming. The possibility of ineffective preverbal semantic monitoring in subjects with MS (e.g. resulting in the production of semantic paraphasias) may be explained by the potential disruption of pathways connecting the temporo-parietal cortex with the caudate nucleus of the basal ganglia and pallido-thalamic fibres associated with MS subcortical white matter demyelination. Lethlean and Murdoch (1994a) speculated that if the cortico-caudate or pallido-thalamic connections are disrupted there may be reduced inhibitory influence of the globus pallidus on the thalamus leading to increased levels of excitation in the anterior language area thereby allowing extraneous inadequately monitored responses to be produced. In their study, the MS subjects were found to produce significantly more semantic paraphasias when compared to the control group. Indeed, according to many researchers, poorly monitored semantic content of language tends to be characterized by semantic paraphasias (Mohr et al., 1975; Cappa and Vignolo, 1979; Alexander and LoVerme, 1980).

Wallesch and Papagno (1988) have proposed that Crosson's (1985) model is too localizationist and that language expression is not necessarily limited to cortical structures. Unlike Crosson's (1985) model, Wallesch and Papagno's (1988) parallel language processing model suggests that language functions are not discretely represented on the cortex in specific one to one relationships but rather that the fundamental functional unit of the brain is a 'module'. Language expressive functions are produced via cortico-striato-pallido-thalamo-cortical loops where the thalamus integrates and gates a possible number of lexical alternatives for production.

Rather than a preverbal semantic monitoring role of the thalamus, as suggested by Crosson (1985), Wallesch and Papagno (1988) have proposed that the thalamus serves an important function in language formulation by not only monitoring language production but also gating cortically transmitted verbal response elements. In addition, they have proposed that the thalamus has an inhibitory influence on the cortex unlike Crosson's (1985) model in which the thalamus has an excitatory influence on the frontal cortical structures. Wallesch and Papagno (1988) describe a 'frontal lobe system' where the head of the caudate nucleus, the globus pallidus, and the ventral thalamus are integrated to influence the frontal cortex. Numerous efferent 'modules' work in parallel and in competition, and the thalamus, under the influence of the basal ganglia, works to integrate or 'gate' the information, choose the desired response, and transmit it to the cortex for production.

The presence of significantly more semantic paraphasias in the MS group compared to the control group observed by Lethlean and Murdoch (1994a) may be explained by a disrupted thalamic gating mechanism in Wallesch and Papagno's (1998) model. Lethlean and Murdoch (1994a) speculated that if thalamo-cortical fibres are partially interrupted, as potentially may occur in MS subcortical demyelination, inappropriate and ineffectively monitored names for a target picture may be released by the frontal cortex. The globus pallidus may attempt to inhibit the thalamus for a correct name; however, due to interruption to the thalamo-cortical fibres, a majority of the gates in the thalamus will be closed. In turn, the cortex will be disinhibited and all parallel circuits containing possible names for the target picture may reach the cortex for a response. Consequently, the name in the module which completes the circuit and reaches the cortex first will be produced. In the absence of effective thalamic gating, the name for the picture which is accessed may or may not be the correct response. Considering that Lethlean and Murdoch (1994a) did not provide confirmation of lesion sites occurring in their MS group, it is suggested that this speculative discussion does promote an explanation worthy of further study.

Researchers examining MS individuals on neuropsychological and neuroradiological measures seem to support the importance of the relationship between the cortical and subcortical structures in the completion of a naming task. Pozzilli, Bastianello et al. (1991), on the basis of MRI, single photon emission computerized tomography, and neuropsychological evaluation (including a test of naming), revealed significant reduction of function in the frontal lobes and left temporal lobe in a group of MS subjects during cognitive tasks. The researchers proposed that decreased activity in the frontal and temporal lobes reflected cortical suppression or deactivation secondary to disconnection from subcortical structures. It is possible that excessive numbers of semantically related naming errors produced by the MS group examined by Lethlean and Murdoch (1994a) may be attributed to an interruption in cortical-subcortical communication, required for normal naming function and which interfered with the subjects' abilities to monitor verbal output and subsequently access words efficiently from the lexicon.

Although a significantly greater mean number of semantic errors were produced by Lethlean and Murdoch's (1994a) MS group when compared to their control group, both groups exhibited similar patterns of semantic errors. It is possible that similar patterns of errors produced by the MS and control groups in Lethlean and Murdoch's (1994a) study may indicate that both groups employ similar strategies to overcome naming deficits. The MS subjects' attempts to describe the target, tallied by Lethlean and Murdoch (1994a) as definitional and vague circumlocutions, may also have reflected a strategy the subjects were using in order to facilitate naming the pictures.

Lethlean and Murdoch (1994a) concluded that the naming deficit in MS may not be solely due to either an impaired semantic system or a disrupted perceptual system. A sub-group of their MS subjects produced perceptual errors in response to naming a picture, which may have been attributed to visual disturbances associated with demyelination of the optic nerve or attentional deficits as suggested by Obler (1983). The lexical semantic accessing hypothesis, however, appeared to explain the remaining semantic errors in their MS group which could not be accounted for by perceptual deficits.

Discourse abilities in multiple sclerosis

Farmakides and Boone (1960) recognized that as persons with MS lose motor control and become physically dependent upon those around them, the ability to communicate effectively becomes increasingly important. Rao (1986) noted that no studies had tried to evaluate the effect of the extensive cognitive deficits in MS on everyday function, while others have raised the critical issue that functional communication skills could be expected to be affected by cognitive deficits (Peyser et al., 1990; Cobble et al., 1991). More recently, Foley et al. (1994) noted that many patients with MS report that word-finding and memory problems decrease their ability to communicate effectively with others. Foley et al. (1994) subsequently published a cognitive-behavioural approach to the treatment of communication deficits. However, effective everyday communication requires not only cognitive, but linguistic skills (Dennis and Lovett, 1990). Foley et al. (1994) neglected to provide empirical support for the patients' anecdotal evidence and also failed to investigate likely cognitive and linguistic underpinnings for the reported communication failures. To obtain a complete picture of communicative abilities in MS, we need to look, not at specific linguistic assessments, but at discourse, a functional measure of communication. According to Ulatowska and Chapman (1989), 'discourse is a unit of language which conveys a message' (p. 299). The success of discourse is dependent upon such factors as lexical, grammatical, pragmatic, and cognitive competence (Dennis and Lovett, 1990). The speaker needs to be able to store events in memory, integrate new and existing knowledge, and retrieve this knowledge (Terrell and Ripich, 1989).

Discourse can take the form of a variety of genres: conversational, narrative, procedural or expository. Different discourse genres place different cognitive and linguistic demands on the individual to plan, organize and convey information. The two most commonly investigated forms of discourse are, in fact, conversation and narrative discourse.

Conversational discourse assessment, though socially valid (Hinckley and Craig, 1992), has certain methodological flaws. Different conversational partners may assume different burdens for maintaining the interaction thus contributing to variability between communicative partners. Topics of discussion may also vary leading to the problem of how to control for content while keeping the interaction natural (Glosser and Deser, 1990). In addition, conversational samples can be time consuming to collect (up to 20 minutes), transcribe and analyse (Chenery and Murdoch, 1994). It is also difficult to judge accuracy because the examiner may not possess the necessary background knowledge to make judgements about the accuracy of conversational content. Furthermore, as the underlying intent is not always clear during a conversation, semantic errors can be underestimated and semantic paraphasias can go undetected (Blanken et al., 1987).

These problems can be overcome with the use of narrative discourse assessment where the researcher has prior knowledge of expected discourse content and is, therefore, able to make judgements about message accuracy (Chenery and Murdoch, 1994). Narrative discourse is more efficient to elicit, transcribe and analyse, and by manipulating the complexity of the stimuli, the amount of information and degree of interpretation required can be changed to produce a hierarchy of tasks. Although more artificial than conversational discourse, narratives can be useful research and clinical tools that allow greater control of variables and, therefore, elicit more comparable discourse samples.

Only two reported studies have attempted to document the spoken narrative abilities of individuals with MS (Wallace and Holmes, 1993; Arnott et al., 1997). Wallace and Holmes (1993) administered a picture description subtest, as part of the Arizona Battery for Communication Disorders of Dementia (ABCD) (Bayles and Tomoeda, 1991), to a group of persons with MS. Similar to the reported findings in closed head injury and right hemisphere damage groups (Ehrlich, 1988; Parsons et al., 1989; Joanette and Goulet, 1990), the MS subjects produced fewer utterances per minute, less complete syntactically correct utterances per minute and a smaller number of information units per utterance than matched controls. However, this was a pilot study involving only four subjects, all with a CP disease course. The study was also designed to test the sensitivity of the ABCD to cognitive/linguistic deficits in MS, and not to document narrative abilities. Nevertheless, by highlighting deficits of informative content and communicative efficiency in narrative discourse, the results of the Wallace and Holmes (1993) study signified that discourse skills in MS warranted further investigation.

In a larger study, Arnott et al. (1997) elicited discourse samples from 47 persons with MS and 47 matched controls in response to computer-generated, animated sequences. In particular, the information conveyed during narrative discourse was analysed by these authors to ascertain whether MS affects a person's ability to effectively plan message content. Within the conceptual level of discourse processing, data were analysed for story schema and informative content. Arnott et al. (1997) reported that the two groups, MS and control, could not be distinguished by measures of the quantity of information conveyed. However, there was a difference in the nature of the information produced by the two groups. The persons with MS produced less essential story information than control subjects, while a tendency for the individuals with MS to produce more incorrect and ambiguous information than controls was also noted. Arnott et al. (1997) postulated that both pragmatic and cognitive skills impact on performance in the narrative genre; hence, deficits in these areas may have contributed to the observed performance deficits. They considered the nature of the discourse deficits observed to be consistent with subcortical plaque damage affecting fibre tracts between and within the cerebral hemispheres. It was concluded by Arnott et al. (1997) that discourse analysis may be sensitive to subtle communication impairments subsequent to MS and prompted them to call for further investigation of discourse abilities in this population.

Chapter 9
Subgroups of multiple sclerosis patients based on language dysfunction

Jennifer B Lethlean and Bruce E Murdoch

Introduction

In earlier chapters of this book it was established that individuals with multiple sclerosis (MS) may present with a range of language impairments, particularly in the area of high-level language function (see Chapters 7 and 8). Group studies have shown that in addition to naming difficulties, word fluency deficits and a reduced ability to repeat sentences, people with MS may also exhibit problems with tasks requiring verbal explanation, verbal reasoning, reconstruction of sentences, definitions of words, and interpretation of absurdities, ambiguities and metaphors. As is the case with other signs and symptoms of MS, however, when examined at an individual level, persons with MS make up a heterogeneous population with respect to language abilities. For instance, examination of the 60 cases of MS studied by Lethlean and Murdoch (1997) on an individual basis, shows that while some of the subjects were linguistically impaired, others performed within normal limits on the language tests administered by those authors. Lethlean and Murdoch (1997) proposed that the variable performance of the MS individuals on the language tests may reflect a combination of variables relating to the disease such as disease course, disease duration, drug treatment, site and number of white matter lesions in the brain etc. Although as a group, variables such as age, education, disease course and disease duration were not related reliably to impaired performance on language tasks in their study, Lethlean and Murdoch (1997) suggested that one or more of these variables may have contributed to the presence of language deficits in individual MS subjects.

An understanding of the different patterns of language impairment exhibited by individuals with MS may be important for a number of theoretical as well as clinical reasons. First, different patterns of performance may relate to site of lesion and may have implications for increased understanding of brain function such as the involvement of subcortical white matter pathways in language processing. Secondly, certain patterns of language dysfunction may contribute to specific difficulties experienced by individuals with MS in their practical, everyday function. For example, the manifestation of a high-level language problem in a person with MS may be indicative of that person's reduced ability to cope in the workplace, particularly in employment situations which require problem-solving, explanation and rationalization through language expression (e.g. as may be required in managerial positions). The need exists, therefore, to investigate and define subgroups of MS patients on the basis of their different patterns of language disability. To this end, the authors of the present chapter have recently analysed the language data collected from the 60 MS subjects investigated by Lethlean and Murdoch (1997), for the presence of subgroups based on language performance. The section below will focus on providing a synthesis of the findings of this analysis.

Language subgroups in multiple sclerosis

To determine the presence of subgroups based on language performance, eight language measures were selected from the language profiles of the 60 individuals with MS described in Chapter 7 and subsequently used in a hierarchical cluster analysis. Personal and medical details of the 60 subjects are listed in Tables 7.2 and 7.3 (see Chapter 7). The eight pre-set language variables included the total Boston Naming Test (BNT) (Kaplan et al., 1983) score, Test of Language Competence (TLC) (Wiig and Secord, 1985) subtests including Understanding Ambiguous Sentences (UAS), Recreating Sentences (RS) and Understanding Metaphoric Expressions (UME), The Word Test (TWT) (Jorgensen et al., 1981) total score, total Wiig-Semel Test of Linguistic Concepts (WST) (Wiig and Semel, 1974) score, and Neurosensory Centre Comprehensive Examination for Aphasia (NCCEA) (Spreen and Benton, 1969) subtests 8 (Word Fluency) and 11 (Token Test). The total test language scores, where all 60 subjects completed the entire test, were included in the cluster as they represented composite measures of the MS subjects' language performance. Subtests 8 and 11 of the NCCEA were also included in the cluster analysis to provide measures of divergent naming and auditory comprehension. The TLC composite score, however, was not included in the cluster analysis because not all subjects attempted the Making Inferences subtest. Therefore, the UAS, RS and UME subtests independently represented the MS subjects' performance on the TLC.

The results of the cluster analysis revealed that the MS subjects could be divided into four subgroups according to the severity of their language impairment, with the four subgroups demonstrating a regular progression in the level of language impairment from one subgroup to another. Subgroup 1 consisted of a single MS subject with a severe language disturbance. Subgroup 2 comprised 8 individuals with MS who demonstrated moderately to severely impaired linguistic abilities, while subgroup 3 included 19 subjects with MS with mild to moderate selectively impaired language functions. The remaining 32 individuals with MS comprised subgroup 4 and presented with essentially normal performances on the selected language tasks. To enable description of the linguistic characteristics of the MS subjects clustered into the four subgroups, each subgroup's mean performance on the eight language variables was compared to the average scores achieved by a group of 60 non-neurologically impaired, matched controls on the same tests. The language characteristics of each subgroup are described below.

Subgroup 1 – Severe pervasive language impairment

Subgroup 1 consisted of one 51-year-old female individual, MS subject 23 (see Table 7.2), who performed consistently below the control group on all eight of the language measures. Subject 23 attained a BNT score of 18, which was 12.4 standard deviations below the controls' mean performance. Her scores on the TLC subtests UAS (score = 7), RS (score = 28) and UME (score = 11) fell 9.3, 18.0 and 9.6 standard deviations, respectively, below the controls' mean scores. In comparison to the controls, subject 23 attained a score of 49 on TWT, which was 11.9 standard deviations below the mean. Subject 23 also performed 13.0 standard deviations below the controls on the WST, attaining a score of 32. The subject's NCCEA scores were compared to that of a normal adult reference population on Form A, which specifies the impaired range of performance as below the 40th percentile (Spreen and Benton, 1969). Her score on subtest 8 (score = 19) was found to reflect impaired word fluency abilities as it fell at the fourth percentile on Form A. A score of 91 on subtest 11 placed subject 23 well below the second percentile for normal adults on Form A, indicating poor auditory comprehension skills.

Subgroup 2 – Moderate to severe language impairment

Eight of the individuals with MS clustered into subgroup 2. On average, the individuals in subgroup 2 attained a BNT score 5.7 standard deviations below the control mean. Performance on the WST reflected a score 6.9 standard deviations lower than the controls' performance average. The mean scores attained by subgroup 2 on TLC subtests UAS, RS and

UME fell 7.3, 15.4 and 6.8 standard deviations respectively below the control means. On TWT and the NCCEA subtests 8 and 11, subgroup 2 performed 11.9, 2.5 and 15.4 standard deviations, respectively, below the control means.

Subgroup 3 – Mild to moderate language impairment

Subgroup 3 consisted of 19 individuals with MS. This group's mean BNT and WST total scores fell 3.9 and 2.2 standard deviations, respectively, below the mean scores for the control group. Subgroup 3 also performed below the control group on the TLC subtests. On the subtests UAS, RS and UME the MS subjects performed 4.32, 8.47 and 4.08 standard deviations, respectively, below the mean scores of the control group. The mean scores achieved on TWT and the NCCEA subtests 8 and 11 fell 5.3, 1.4 and 9.6 standard deviations, respectively, below the average performances of the control group.

Subgroup 4 – Essentially normal language abilities

The last group, subgroup 4, consisted of 32 MS subjects who attained marginally lower scores than the control group on all of the language measures used in the cluster analysis. This group's mean BNT and WST scores fell less than one standard deviation below the control group's mean scores. The MS subjects' average performance on the TLC subtests UAS, RS and UME reflected scores 2.0, 2.8 and 1.7 standard deviations below the control group's mean performance on these language tasks. The MS subjects also attained slightly lower scores than the control group on TWT and the NCCEA subtests 8 and 11 reflecting scores 2.3, 1.0 and 3.7 standard deviations, respectively, below the control means.

Factors influencing language abilities in multiple sclerosis subgroups

A number of subject variables such as age, education level, disease duration, disease course, the degree of visual impairment, physical status, medications, residential status, extent and site of white matter lesions, and cognitive status may contribute to the varied degree of language impairment observed in the MS subgroups described above. Consequently, an examination of the characteristics which may have contributed to the differential language abilities of the four MS subgroups was carried out.

Peyser et al. (1980) clustered 55 MS subjects according to age, sex, education level, disease state, duration of disease, physical disability, manual dexterity, and abstract reasoning. The cluster analysis identified six different groups, four of which were characterized by their age, physical disability, disease duration, and cognitive status (Peyser et al., 1980). For example, cluster 1 in Peyser et al.'s (1980) study consisted of patients with the longest illness duration, greatest physical difficulty and cognitive impairment. It is possible that this cluster was formed by subjects with similar characteristics to the MS individuals with substantial language deficits that comprised subgroup 2 in our analysis described above.

Older adults have been found to demonstrate an age-related decrement in their use of effortful information processing of words and sentences (Byrd, 1988). In addition, age and, to a lesser but significant extent, educational level have been correlated with cognitive and neuropsychological test performance (Goldstein and Shelly, 1975; Finlayson et al., 1977). Statistical comparisons of the demographic variables of subgroups 2, 3 and 4 identified in our analysis, however, revealed that age and education did not serve to differentiate the subgroups. This finding supports the results of naming studies where no significant correlations have been identified between the BNT total score and age and education (Van Gorp et al., 1986; Nicholas et al., 1989).

Disease duration has been reported as a variable which may contribute to the diverse performance of MS individuals on cognitive and associated language tasks (e.g. Ron et al., 1991; Mendozzi et al., 1993). As in the case of age and education, however, statistical analysis revealed that there was no difference in the average disease duration of the individuals with MS comprising the subgroups identified in our analysis. The more linguistically impaired individuals were not necessarily the subjects who had been diagnosed with MS for a longer period of time.

Lethlean and Murdoch (1994b) reported that naming deficits tend to be more severe in those MS individuals with a chronically progressive (CP) disease course. The proportions of individuals with a CP disease course in subgroups 2, 3 and 4, however, were found to be statistically similar although all eight subjects with MS in subgroup 2, which comprised individuals with substantial linguistic impairments, presented with a CP type of MS.

One of the commonly reported symptoms of MS is unilateral or bilateral optic nerve dysfunction (Rao, 1986). Consequently, subjects with MS have been found to perform poorly on visuospatial tasks (Caine et al., 1986; Huber et al., 1987; Van den Burg et al., 1987; Beatty et al., 1988). According to Rao (1986), primary sensorimotor deficits and/or focal disruption of visuoperceptual, visuospatial and visuoconstructive processes are potentially confounding variables in neuropsychological assessments of individuals with MS. In the study carried out by the present authors, however, with the exception of the BNT and the NCCEA subtest 11 (Token Test), it is suggested that visual impairment is unlikely to have contributed to poor performance on the language measures employed in the correlation as the tests did not require maximal visual acuity. Indeed, examination of the subjects in the MS subgroups revealed that there were similar proportions of visually impaired subjects in all three of the subgroups comprised of more than one individual. It is proposed that visual impairment did not serve to differentiate the MS subgroups identified in our study. However, further research incorporating tests of visual processing is required to determine the influence of visual deficits on linguistic task performance.

The severity of physical disability and the requirement for institutionalized care also did not appear to differ among the MS subgroups identified by the present authors, as similar proportions of wheelchair dependent and institutionalized MS individuals were identified in the various subgroups. It is suggested, however, that the overall severity of MS, as could be determined through measures of functional systems including pyramidal, cerebellar, brain stem, sensory, bowel and bladder, visual, cerebral-total, cerebral-mentation (Kurtze, 1983b), and associated dependency on others in daily living tasks, may have characterized the subgroups. The overall severity of MS may have been reflected in the performance of the MS subjects on the high-level language tests. Further discussion of this suggestion, however, is not possible at this time as quantitative neurological assessments of MS severity were not carried out in our study.

Various medications, used in the treatment of MS symptoms, may affect speech and higher level cognitive functions (Hodgson, 1993). In the present study, individuals with MS were reportedly on drug regimes including psychoactive drugs such as benzodiazepines (e.g. valium and mogadon) for muscle spasms and anxiety control, corticosteroids (e.g. prednisone) for immunosuppression to reduce clinical exacerbations, tricyclic antidepressants (e.g. tryptanol and tofranil), and antiepileptics (e.g. dilantin and tegretol). According to Hodgson (1993), benzodiazepines, tricyclic antidepressants and antiepileptics may disrupt cognitive processing and may contribute to word retrieval difficulties. It is possible that the side effects of psychoactive drugs may have contributed to poorer naming performance by the linguistically impaired MS subjects in subgroups 2 and 3 when compared to the subjects in subgroup 4 with near normal high-level language abilities and the control group. While researchers have suggested that psychoactive medication may contribute to mild memory impairment in MS (Rao et al., 1984), other authors have proposed that medications cannot explain the severely impaired performances on cognitive tasks (Rao et al., 1984; Heaton et al., 1985). Indeed, an examination of our MS subjects revealed similar proportions of individuals on medications in the various subgroups identified by us on the basis of language abilities. The individual effects of type and dose of medications, however, were not examined by us and consequently it is suggested that the possible effects of specific medications on the language abilities of individuals with MS be the subject of future investigations.

Considering the proposed interdependent relationship of cognition and language (Bayles and Boone, 1982) it is suggested that the MS subjects in the linguistically impaired subgroups may have exhibited greater neuropsychological deficits. Indeed, cognitive deficits associated with diffuse white matter lesions and the onset of dementia may have contributed, in part, to the distribution of the MS cases into the subgroups. It is proposed, however, that differentiating cognitive and linguistic abilities in the MS population would be difficult considering the sensory and motor difficulties associated with the disease. Even performance on a non-linguistic cognitive assessment could be potentially confounded by the MS subjects' visual and upper body fine motor difficulties. Irrespective of the basis for the language impairment (linguistic or cognitive or both), which could not be determined from our findings, the deficits manifested as poor performances on the language tests. More detailed research is required to determine the relationship between the cognitive and linguistic deficits in MS.

There have been a number of studies that have documented significant correlations between the site and extent of MS white matter lesions apparent on neuroradiological examination and MS subjects' performance on neuropsychological assessments (e.g. Izquierdo et al., 1991; Swirsky-Sacchetti et al., 1992). Forebrain lesion load has been found to be closely related to measures of cognitive and memory impairment in chronically progressive MS subjects (Rao, Leo et al., 1989). Hemispheric lesions on magnetic resonance imaging (MRI) may be a useful tool in predicting memory and learning impairment (Izquierdo et al., 1991; Swirsky-Sacchetti et al., 1992). Other researchers, however, have questioned the reliability of the correlation between cognitive difficulties and MRI findings (Huber et al., 1992). Huber et al. (1992) found no significant differences between MS groups with normal or mild and moderate overall cognitive impairment on any MRI measures. Subjects with severe cognitive deficits, however, presented with corpus callosum atrophy and larger lesions regardless of location. More specifically, the researchers proposed that atrophy of the corpus callosum reflected fronto-temporal and parieto-occipital dysfunction, which may result in generalized cognitive impairment (Huber et al., 1992). Performance on the neuropsychological assessment, however, was not systematically related to the distribution of white matter lesions (Huber et al., 1992). For example, Huber et al. (1992) found that there was no difference in the relationship between verbal or non-verbal ability and lesion areas in the left and right cerebral hemispheres. It is possible that the language deficits identified in the MS subjects examined by the present authors may relate to site and number of focal areas of demyelination in the central nervous system; however, definitive answers can be arrived at only following correlations of quantitative measures of lesion load on MRI and scores on language tasks. Although objective neuroradiological findings were not available for all of the subjects examined in our study, it is hypothesized that the linguistically impaired MS subjects in subgroups 2 and 3 may have experienced more extensive subcortical demyelination when compared to the MS subjects in subgroup 4 who had relatively intact high-level language abilities. Therefore, potential white matter disconnections interrupting cortical and subcortical communication may explain the significantly more severe language deficits exhibited by the MS subjects in subgroups 2 and 3. Further research is required, however, to consider the relationship between location and number of white matter lesions in MS and performance on high-level language and naming tasks.

In summary, although comparison of the various language subgroups on individual subject variables (i.e. age, education level, disease duration, visual impairment, physical disability and drug regimen) suggested that these variables alone did not contribute to the observed differences in language abilities, it is possible that the combined effect of the variables contributed to the severity of the language impairment. It is suggested that the substantially language impaired individuals in subgroups 2 and 3 comprised MS subjects with a combination of associated deficits. It is speculated that those individuals who were older, less educated, had a lengthy disease duration, were visually impaired, in a wheelchair, and taking psychoactive drugs were more likely to perform poorly on the language tasks. In addition, subject variables such as site and number of lesions and an actual measure of disease severity may have contributed to the way the subjects clustered into subgroups. Indeed, one would expect that those MS subjects with more lesions localized in the subcortical white matter pathways connecting left cortical and subcortical structures would present with more severely impaired performances on the language tests. It is likely that those subjects with more extensive demyelination would present with more severe symptoms of MS. Further conclusions concerning the basis for the language deficits and the distribution of the MS subjects into the clustered subgroups, however, can only be based on further detailed examination of relevant demographic and MS disease variables, including comprehensive neurological, neuroradiological and neuropsychological assessments, in relation to language performance.

Variability of language abilities in multiple sclerosis

The finding that individuals with MS may be subgrouped according to their language abilities highlights the heterogeneous nature of language impairment in the MS population. Indeed, it was established in the previous section of this chapter that the language abilities of persons with MS may vary from severe linguistic impairment to language abilities within normal limits. Further, the MS cases described above illustrate the range of language profiles that clinicians may encounter in their clients with MS. This section of the present chapter will examine in detail the language abilities of a representative sample of individuals with MS based on their performance on the high-level language test battery administered by Lethlean and Murdoch (1997). In addition, the language deficits identified in each subject will be discussed in relation to a contemporary model of subcortical language processing (Wallesch and Papagno, 1988).

The individuals with MS to be discussed were selected from the four MS subgroups based on language abilities described earlier in this chapter. The single individual with MS that comprised subgroup 1 was not selected for discussion here, as her performance on the language tasks was outlined previously (see section relating to language subgroups in MS above). Those MS cases selected for discussion here were chosen on the basis that they were considered representative of the differentially impaired language groups. Subjects 12, 16, 24 and 26 were chosen to represent subgroup 2, reflecting substantial language deficits. From subgroup 3, which included cases with selective impairment of more complex cognitive/linguistic skills, subjects 4, 11, 20 and 41 were chosen for discussion, while subjects 21, 40 and 46 were selected as representative of subgroup 4, reflecting subjects with near normal language abilities. The demographic and disease characteristics of the selected subjects with MS are presented in Tables 7.2 and 7.3 (see Chapter 7). The language tests administered to each subject are the same as those used by Lethlean and Murdoch (1997) and included the NCCEA, BNT, TLC, TWT and the WST. For the purpose of discussion in the present chapter, the performances of the selected MS subjects on the high-level language tests were compared with normative test data wherever available. In those instances where normative data were not available, the scores achieved by the subjects with MS were compared to those of a matched group of non-neurologically impaired controls.

Each MS subject's score on the NCCEA was compared with the NCCEA Profile Form A for normal adults (Spreen and Benton, 1969). Scores falling below the 40th percentile on the language subtests were considered as impaired according to Spreen and Benton's (1969) stipulated criteria for the NCCEA. The MS subjects' performances on the BNT were reported as impaired or normal according to the criteria provided by Nicholas et al. (1989) where a score below 48 reflects impaired naming. Limited adult normative data was available for the TLC, TWT and WST; therefore the scores achieved by the MS subjects on these tests were compared to the control group in terms of standard deviations above or below the mean.

Case reports – Language subgroup 2 (substantive language impairment)

Case report 1 (Subject 12)

Subject 12 was a 48-year-old female with 12 years of schooling who reported that her first symptoms of MS occurred at the age of 22 when her foot began dragging as she walked. At that time, she also went temporarily blind in one eye. Later the same year, following a series of neurological and radiological tests, she was diagnosed with MS by a neurologist. Immediately after the diagnosis of MS was made, the subject's symptoms went into remission. Eight years later she had a relapse and then experienced further remissions and exacerbations every two years. Since the age of 40, however, she had experienced gradual deterioration of her condition, reflecting a chronically progressive (CP) disease course.

At the time when the language assessment was completed, subject 12 exhibited intact abilities on the simple expressive tasks of the NCCEA, including visual naming, left-hand tactile naming, reading and writing. Relatively low scores were attained by subject 12, however, on the tasks assessing repetition of sentences, and repetition and reversal of digit sequences.

Further examination of subject 12's high-level language skills revealed that she presented with areas of impaired expressive and receptive language functioning. She demonstrated considerable word-finding difficulties on the NCCEA as indicated by her production of significantly fewer names on the word fluency task when compared to the control group, and below normal scores on TWT tasks requiring her to access synonyms and antonyms. Her right-handed tactile naming of simple objects was also found to be impaired. Poor verbal explanation skills were evident when the subject attempted to describe the use of simple objects, define specific words, and explain absurd sentences, syntactically and lexically ambiguous sentences and metaphorical expressions. For example, on task C of TWT, subject 12 provided an inadequate explanation 'That's ridiculous, you usually do sleep all night' for the absurd sentence 'Judy was exhausted from sleeping all night long'.

Although subject 12 attained a maximum score on the limited NCCEA measure of sentence construction, she demonstrated relatively impaired abilities when asked to complete the more complex sentence construction subtest of the TLC, which employed more linguistic constraints. Some of the sentences she created tended to be unacceptable syntactic, semantic and/or pragmatic productions. For example, when requested to formulate a sentence with the words 'difficult', 'now' and 'nonetheless', in response to a picture of people moving house, the subject used all three words and created the grammatically awkward sentence 'Nonetheless the last furniture had to go now being difficult.' Other responses consisted of grammatically and syntactically appropriate sentences, but did not include all three of the words provided.

While the subject had difficulties with some of the verbal explanation tasks, TWT and the TLC revealed that she was able to select an appropriate response where multiple choice information was provided. Indeed, her performances on the tasks requiring her to select a word not belonging to a category, make inferences, and select matching metaphors were relatively unimpaired.

Subject 12 attained a score on the Token Test of the NCCEA which reflected intact auditory comprehension abilities. In contrast, receptive language difficulties were demonstrated by the subject on the more complex WST. Indeed, she presented with significantly impaired syntactical logical operations when processing comparative, temporal, passive and spatial concepts. The difficulties the subject had while explaining the lexically or syntactically ambiguous sentences and metaphors on the TLC may have also been related to poor comprehension abilities.

Case report 2 (Subject 16)

Subject 16 was a 76-year-old woman with 10 years of schooling. She reported that her initial symptoms of MS were double vision and clumsiness at the age of 42 which resolved after a few months. Exacerbation of her symptoms later the same year, subsequent hospitalization and neurological testing resulted in the diagnosis of MS. Between the ages of 42 and 53, subject 16 reported a relapsing-remitting (RR) disease course with intermittent sensory and physical MS symptoms. Since the age of 54, however, her symptoms had progressively worsened, reflecting a chronically progressive course of the disease.

At the time of language testing subject 16 was wheelchair dependent, and able to transfer and manage self-care activities. When asked about her speech, she reported occasional slurring of her words especially at the end of the day when she was tired. She presented, however, with perceptibly normal speech when completing the language assessments. Subject 16 demonstrated competent abilities on the language tasks of the NCCEA requiring her to name visually, describe the use of simple objects, and name tactually using her right hand. Her communication skills, enabling her to repeat sentences, repeat and reverse sequences of digits, read, write and articulate, were also within normal limits.

Considerably impaired expressive and receptive language abilities were identified when subject 16 was assessed on TWT and the TLC. Her poor naming abilities identified using the BNT score on the BNT compromised her word fluency abilities, and difficulty retrieving synonyms and antonyms was suggestive of word-finding difficulties. In addition, the subject's tactile naming abilities using her left hand were found to be impaired. Subject 16's inadequate performance on a number of verbal explanation and linguistic tasks was suggestive of deficient expressive high-level language function. Indeed, she provided poor explanations for absurd, ambiguous (syntactically or lexically) and metaphorical sentences, had difficulty providing definitions for lexical items, and demonstrated a compromised ability to explain associations between words. For example, in subtest 1 of the TLC, subject 16 failed to detect the ambiguity in the syntactically ambiguous item 'The man was sure that the duck was ready to eat' and proposed two similar explanations 'It was cooked' and 'It'd been plucked.'

Problems were also experienced by subject 16 when she attempted to incorporate three words into a sentence on the TLC, whereas she was able to complete the simple sentence construction task on the NCCEA without time constraints. She tended to produce sentences on the TLC that were grammatically, semantically and pragmatically inappropriate and which did not always include all the words required for completion of the task. For example, when given a stimulus picture of 'in front of the school' and the words 'crowded', 'drive' and 'if', she responded 'The bus was crowded with school children if we wait for the next bus'. Overall on TWT and the TLC tasks, she demonstrated deficient rationalization and cognitive/linguistic processing skills.

Subject 16 had difficulty choosing the correct word which did not belong from four lexical items in a common category on task A of TWT. In addition, she was unable to explain the reason for her choice in relation to the category of the other three words. For instance, when given the words 'lemonade', 'milk', 'icecream' and 'cheese', she selected the word 'milk' and gave the reason 'because it's good for you'. She also had problems making inferences and choosing a matching metaphor when given a selection of four. During the testing sessions, subject 16 appeared to have difficulty understanding the instructions for some of TWT and the TLC subtests. Instructions had to be repeated several times and examples provided before she could complete the tasks.

Subject 16 was found to perform poorly on the comprehension measures of the language test battery when compared to normative data. She attained scores below normal limits on the Token Test of the NCCEA and made significantly more errors relative to the control subjects when processing passive concepts and familial relationships on the WST.

Case report 3 (Subject 24)

Subject 24 was a 59-year-old female with 10 years of schooling. She was diagnosed with MS at the age of 26 and records from her medical chart reported that she had experienced intermittent diplopia since the age of 17. In her early twenties she presented with weakness and numbness in her right arm and leg; however, this resolved after a week. Following sensation changes and a feeling of being 'weak all over', at the age of 26, she was admitted to hospital and MS was provisionally diagnosed. At the age of 44 she needed to use sticks for walking and then became wheel-chair dependent in her late forties, requiring nursing assistance for daily living tasks. The diagnosis of a CP type of MS was confirmed by neuro-logical and radiological assessments at the age of 57 years.

At the time of diagnosis, subject 24 presented with slurring of speech, episodic facial neuralgia, problems with bladder retention, weakness and clumsiness of hands and intermittent parasthesias, and heaviness and numbness in her legs. She had mild to moderate pyramidal weakness of her upper limbs with a moderate intention tremor. An assessment of her lower limbs revealed decreased muscle tone, slight wasting and severe weakness in both limbs resulting in an inability to walk. For both upper and lower limbs her joint position and vibration senses were absent. Touch and pain perceptions, however, were normal.

A visual examination revealed a normal left optic disc, an atrophic right optic disc, an absent right corneal reflex, ataxic nystagmus, vertical nystagmus looking down, and horizontal and rotational nystagmus looking up. Brain stem auditory evoked response (AER) assessments identified a marginal delay in the right ear indicating hearing loss or demyelination. The AER findings in the left ear were reported as consis-tent with brainstem dysfunction. Cerebrospinal examination revealed oligoclonal bands, a mildly elevated glucose level of 5.3 (normal range 2.5 to 5.0) and non-reactive cryptococcal antigen testing. Electrolyte, urea, creatine and liver function tests were normal. An electroencephalogram (EEG) revealed some excess slow wave activity post-centrally over both cerebral hemispheres. The EEG findings were reported to be related to minor subcortical injury. A computerized tomography (CT) scan performed and interpreted by a radiologist showed generalized prominence of the cerebral sulci and fissures, and prominences of the basal cisterns and lateral, third and fourth ventricles in keeping with generalized cerebral atrophy. No focal lesions were demonstrated. The medical chart reported that an MRI scan showed multiple areas of increased signal on T_2 weighted scans. Further details of the MRI scans, however, were not available.

Although at the time of language assessment the subject presented with a mild to moderate dysarthria, her speech was judged as intelligible by the examiner. The language tests showed that Subject 24 exhibited intact visual naming and was able to describe the use of simple objects as indicated by her scores on the NCCEA. She also attained scores within normal limits on the sentence repetition, digit repetition, reading and articulation subtests of the NCCEA. She presented, however, with an impaired ability to reverse sequences of digits, impaired writing skills, and compromised right and left tactile naming abilities.

Examination of more complex language functions revealed that subject 24 also had some deficits in the production and comprehension of language. Although the subject was able to name the objects in the NCCEA, significant word-finding deficits were identified on higher level tests of word retrieval. Indeed, impaired scores were attained by subject 24 on the BNT and comparatively few lexical items were generated on the word fluency subtest. In addition, she had problems providing synonyms and antonyms for a series of words. For example, in task D of TWT, she gave the incorrect word 'welcome' as an antonym for the word 'dangerous'.

Subject 24 presented with relatively deficient verbal expressive skills as she had difficulty explaining absurdities and metaphors, and gave inadequate definitions for specific words. For example, an inadequate definition provided for the word 'stadium' on task E of TWT was 'gathering of people'. In this example, she failed to include the critical elements of place and an appropriate activity.

Although subject 24 could adequately construct sentences on the NCCEA, she had significant problems recreating sentences requiring the inclusion of more complex lexical items. Her responses tended to be awkward and grammatically incorrect and for some items she failed to incorporate all the target words in the sentences. For example, using the words 'job', 'but' and 'easy', in the context of a house renovation, she created the inaccurate sentence 'Carrying the rubbish could be the easiest wouldn't it?' Although subject 24 demonstrated the ability to provide a single meaning for some of the syntactically or lexically ambiguous sentences, she failed to process, plan and construct a second interpretation.

While subject 24 had difficulty verbally explaining some of her responses she demonstrated the ability to select, for some items, an appropriate single answer when given a multiple-choice type of question. She was able to categorize vocabulary items according to their class name and semantic features (e.g. size and colour) but had problems verbalizing why a selected item did not belong to the category of the other three. Even though the subject provided poor explanations for metaphors, she was able to select an accurate meaning for most items, from a choice of four. When making inferences, however, she tended to choose one correct and one inappropriate answer from a selection of four. Assessments of receptive language function revealed that subject 24 had comprehension difficulties on the Token Test of the NCCEA when compared to the control group. Her poor logico-grammatical processing of spatial concepts was also evident on the WST.

Case report 4 (Subject 26)

Subject 26, a 47-year-old female with six years of education, was admitted to hospital at the age of 42 years for investigation of a four-year history of gait disturbance. She had noted an increased unsteadiness on her feet and discomfort in the right occipital area of her neck, but there was no associated weakness or numbness in her legs and her arm function was normal. The only other significant history was that of occasional difficulty in finding words and reported memory deterioration.

Neurological examination revealed normal power and tone of the subject's limbs although her gait was mildly ataxic. Deep tendon reflexes were brisk in the lower limbs and plantar responses were equivalent bilaterally. Sensation testing was normal for all modalities. Visual and cranial nerve examinations and bowel and bladder function were also normal. Cerebellar assessments revealed no past pointing or intention tremor. Further initial examinations of the subject's other systems were normal.

A psychological assessment using the Wechsler Adult Intelligence Scale (WAIS) revealed that scores were uniformly low. Her full scale intelligence quotient was 76 (borderline performance). On a simple visual recognition task her performance was variable with failures on simple items and passes on more complex ones. Verbal fluency was poor, as she scored below the fourth percentile. A mild to moderate impairment of memory both for verbally and visually presented new learning material was indicated with a memory quotient of 89 (low average performance). Motor control was poor at times and she could not fluidly co-ordinate the movements of her hands on a task of reciprocal motor co-ordination. A frontal type dyspraxia was postulated.

Electrolytes, liver function tests, thyroid function tests, blood tests, chest X-ray and electrocardiogram (ECG) were all normal. Cerebrospinal examination revealed no oligoclonal bands, normal glucose, a normal protein IgG/Albium ratio and a IgG index in the normal range. An EEG revealed a regular alpha rhythm with no focal or epileptogenic features present. Visual evoked responses were performed on both eyes and were found to be normal with no evidence of demyelination. A possible differential diagnosis including CP MS, a high cervical lesion causing cord compression, or a normal pressure hydrocephalus was proposed. A myelogram and a CT scan of the upper cervical spine, however, were found to be within normal limits excluding a high cervical lesion. All the negative investigations indicated an unclear aetiology of the gait and neuropsychological disturbances.

An MRI scan taken near the time of the language assessment reported numerous areas of high signal intensity scattered throughout the white matter of the centrum semiovale and periventricular region, confirming a diagnosis of MS (see Figure 9.1). Plaques were also found to be evident in the cerebellar hemispheres but there was no evidence of significant mass effect. At the time of language assessment subject 26 presented with perceptibly normal speech but she reported some difficulty remembering addresses and phone numbers.

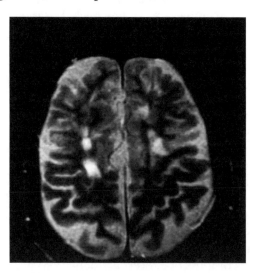

Figure 9.1 A magnetic resonance image showing areas of high signal intensity scattered throughout the white matter of the centrum semiovale and periventricular region (T_2 weighted image with spin echo sequence TE/TR = 85/3000) for multiple sclerosis subject 26

The language tests showed that subject 26 was able to name simple objects using visual and tactile information. She described the use of objects adequately and performed similarly to the control subjects on the tasks requiring her to repeat sentences, repeat and reverse digits, read, write, and articulate.

Examination of subject 26's performances on measures of high-level language abilities also revealed some expressive and receptive deficits. She presented with word-finding difficulties on the more sensitive measure of confrontation naming, namely the BNT. In addition, she demonstrated impaired vocabulary skills when required to access synonyms and antonyms on TWT and her ability to generate lexical items on the word fluency subtest of the NCCEA was impaired. Language deficits were identified on verbal explanation tasks, as subject 26 had problems explaining absurd sentences, syntactically ambiguous sentences and metaphors. For example, in the situation 'Two students moving to a new town' presented in the TLC, subject 26 incorrectly interpreted the metaphor 'There is rough sailing ahead for us' as 'They're really battling'; however, she was able to identify the correct match 'We will be facing a hard road' from a choice of four. She also provided poor definitions for the vocabulary items in TWT and responded with inadequate verbal explanations as to why a word did not belong to a group of four words. For example, on task A of TWT, she accurately identified the word 'light' from the other words 'Doorbell', 'siren', and 'whistle', but provided the inaccurate explanation 'you turn it off and on' for her choice.

Although subject 26 attained a maximum score on the sentence construction subtest of the NCCEA, she had difficulty creating sentences using the predetermined context and more complex vocabulary items which were stipulated by the TLC. The sentences she created tended to be semantically and syntactically impaired. In addition, she failed to use each of the three words required for each response. Subject 26 demonstrated the ability to generate a possible conclusion to a specified event but failed to generate a second viable inference for the TLC task.

Subject 26 also demonstrated some receptive language difficulties on the high-level language tasks when compared to the control group. She exhibited relatively mild deficits on the Token Test of the NCCEA and had mild difficulties comprehending spatial concepts on the WST.

Case reports – Language subgroup 3 (Selective high-level language impairment)

Case report 5 (Subject 4)

Subject 4 was a 44-year-old male with 11 years of schooling. A case history provided by the subject revealed that he experienced his first symptoms of

MS, including double vision, at the age of 36. The results of extensive neurological testing the same year indicated the presence of MS. Further details of these assessments, however, were not available for discussion. Since diagnosis, his vision and physical condition had steadily deteriorated, reflecting a CP course of the disease. For three years prior to the language assessment he had been dependent on an automatic wheelchair for mobility and had required assistance at home for daily living skills.

Subject 4 presented with perceptibly normal speech at the time of the language assessment. His persisting visual difficulties, however, appeared to interfere with some of the language tests. Therefore, the influence of his visual problems on his performance in the tests will be considered in the discussion of his test results.

Subject 4 failed to complete the auditory comprehension, reading and writing tasks of the NCCEA and the Making Inferences subtest of the TLC. The remaining language assessments on the NCCEA revealed that he was able to describe the use of objects, repeat sentences and articulate single words. His ability to categorize vocabulary items according to class name, function, size, shape, colour, quality and composition on TWT was intact. In addition, he was able to verbalize the reason the selected item did not belong to the category from a choice of four words. Impaired performances, however, were identified on tasks requiring the subject to repeat and reverse sequences of digits.

Further assessment of subject 4's expressive linguistic skills and comprehension abilities revealed below normal functioning relative to the control group's average performances on the same tasks. He presented with poor word-finding abilities on the naming tasks. Indeed, this was indicated by his production of visual misnamings on the simple items of the NCCEA and his poor performance on the more complex items of the BNT. Both left- and right-handed tactile naming were impaired. Reduced word fluency scores and poor performances on the synonym and antonym tasks of TWT appeared to be indicative of a compromised lexical system.

Subject 4 also had difficulties with some expressive language tasks as indicated by his performance on TWT and the TLC. His verbal explanations of absurd sentences, interpretations of syntactically ambiguous sentences, and his attempts to define words, were inadequate according to the testing criteria. For example, in task F of TWT, requiring multiple meanings of lexical items, for the word 'change', he responded: 'you change your clothes every day' and 'you change to a better environment' which both reflected the same meaning 'to alter'. On the subtest requiring interpretation of metaphorical expressions, subject 4 demonstrated the ability to express the meanings of the metaphors but had difficulty choosing the matching metaphor from a selection of four.

Subject 4 attained a low score on the NCCEA sentence construction subtest which was attributed to the response lag after which he formulated an appropriate sentence. In the TLC sentence construction task, the subject demonstrated the ability to create a holistically acceptable sentence but failed to use all three words in a single sentence.

The high-level language assessments also revealed some evidence of comprehension deficits. Subject 4 attained low scores on the Token Test of the NCCEA and had some difficulties processing the passive and familial concepts on the WST.

Case report 6 (Subject 11)

Subject 11, a 60-year-old woman with 12 years of education reported that, at the age of 48, she first experienced MS symptoms including sensation changes, clumsiness, intermittent hearing loss and visual disturbances. Neurological testing was carried out when she was 50, at which time a diagnosis of CP MS was made. The medical records of her test results, however, were not available for perusal. Since diagnosis, subject 11 reported that, although she remains independently mobile and self-caring, her mobility had been gradually deteriorating.

At the time of language assessment the subject presented with perceptibly normal speech. She reported that although her speech is occasionally quicker and more hesitant, she has no difficulty thinking of words in conversation. The language assessments revealed that Subject 11 exhibited intact performances on simple visual naming, tactile naming, and description of use tasks as indicated by her scores on the NCCEA. Her reading, writing and articulatory abilities were all within normal limits. Normal scores were also achieved on measures of sentence repetition, digit repetition and digit reversal.

Assessments of high-level language revealed that subject 11 performed poorly on some expressive and receptive tasks relative to the control group. Although intact visual naming was identified on the NCCEA, word-finding difficulties were evident, as she attained an impaired level score on the BNT. Competent lexical accessing abilities were demonstrated when she was required to generate items on the NCCEA word fluency tasks and provide synonyms and antonyms on TWT.

Subject 11 presented with some poor expressive language functions as indicated by a compromised ability to provide definitions for words and construct sentences. For example, when required to produce multiple meanings for the word 'chest' on task F of TWT, she provided two responses 'box' and 'glory chest' which reflected the same inherent meaning. Although she was able to produce semantically, syntactically and pragmatically intact sentences, her word count was reduced. That is, she had difficulty planning the response using all three words to be provided in a single sentence. This finding was in contrast to her maximum score on the sentence construction subtest of the NCCEA. Further examination of her high-level language abilities revealed that the subject was able to provide a single interpretation of ambiguous sentences but had difficulty generating a second meaning which explained the lexical or syntactical ambiguity. On the remaining expressive high-level language tasks, subject 11 performed similarly to the control group. She was able to explain absurd sentences and metaphors adequately and make appropriate inferences following the presentation of a short story.

Although the NCCEA measure of auditory comprehension indicated that subject 11 had mildly impaired receptive language abilities, the more complex measure of comprehension, the WST, revealed relatively intact functions.

Case report 7 (Subject 20)

Subject 20 was a 57-year-old male with 10 years of education. His first symptoms of MS appeared at age 21 and included reduced strength, intermittent sensory changes and fainting episodes. At the age of 39 he experienced retrobulbar neuritis, was hospitalized and underwent a series of tests resulting in the diagnosis of CP MS.

An MRI scan taken near to the time of language testing revealed multiple focal areas of increased signal intensity seen throughout the white matter of both cerebral hemispheres, particularly in a periventricular distribution (see Figure 9.2). All of the intracranial cerebrospinal fluid spaces were of generous proportions. The cortical sulci were prominent, suggesting a degree of cerebral atrophy.

Subject 20 completed a psychological assessment at age 55 years. At this time he reported that he had gradually developed a tendency to avoid work and complained of fatigue. The results of the assessments revealed that the subject had an average level of intellectual efficiency and memory function. He performed at an average level, reflected by approximate percentile levels, in the areas of general informational resources, attention span, vocabulary, comprehension, abstract reasoning ability, recognition of social sequence in pictorial representation, and analysing and synthesizing ability. His ability to distinguish between essential and inessential detail, and his fine visuomotor coordination corresponded with low average function. Recognition of part-to-whole relationships reflected high average performance and his concentration abilities were considered as far superior. Personal infor-

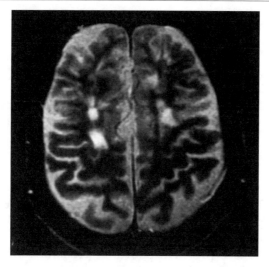

Figure 9.2 A magnetic resonance image showing multiple focal areas of increased signal intensity seen throughout the white matter of both cerebral hemispheres, particularly in a periventricular distribution (T_2 weighted image with spin echo sequence TE/TR = 85/3000) for multiple sclerosis subject 20

mation was consistently given and taken to be reliable but visual recall was found to be unreliable. Knowledge of current events, orientation for time, place and person, mental control and associate learning ability were adequate, but logical sequential recall was only marginally adequate. Overall, his status was considered by the psychologist as consistent with a level of general cognitive deterioration. He was also found to be experiencing moderate depression. On the basis of the psychological assessment, early retirement was recommended.

Psychological retesting two years later revealed further cognitive deterioration when compared to the previous results. In particular, subject 20's verbal IQ score indicated the most loss in function. His attention and concentration span scores had dropped from the 98th percentile to the 22nd percentile and his comprehension level had dropped from the 31st to the 14th percentile. His planning and clerical abilities had also deteriorated considerably. Short-term memory loss was also evident and corresponded with the subject's reported loss in confidence in his memory capacity. The psychologist's report indicated that the subject's work performance would be negatively affected by compromised concentration and memory, poor clerical abilities, depression and an increased level of fatigue.

At the time of language assessment the subject presented with perceptibly normal speech. Subject 20 attained normal scores on the simple visual and tactile naming tasks of the NCCEA. His description of object use, sentence repetition, digit repetition and reversal skills were also intact.

More complex measures of expressive and receptive language function revealed that subject 20 performed poorly on some subtests of TWT and the TLC. Although he presented with intact visual naming on the NCCEA, word-finding difficulties were identified on his BNT performance. He also attained relatively low scores when required to identify synonyms and antonyms on TWT and retrieve lexical items on the NCCEA word fluency task.

The high-level language tasks requiring verbal expression revealed that subject 20 had difficulty defining single words. For example, the inadequate definition the subject gave for the word 'elevator' was 'a mode of transport'. For this item he failed to include the critical elements of motion (e.g. up and down) and place (e.g. building, floor to floor). Subject 20 also provided poor interpretations for metaphorical expressions but was able to select the appropriate meaning when given a choice of four. While the subject was able to choose a correct inference from a selection of four which concluded a story, he failed to generate an alternative situational script. Although he could construct simple sentences on the NCCEA, he appeared to have more difficulty constructing sentences using the criterion specified by the TLC. He produced a number of non-sentences and syntactically and semantically deviant sentences in an attempt to include all three words in his responses. Relatively poor categorization abilities were also identified when he selected the inappropriate word from a group of four on task A of TWT. Intact expressive language abilities were identified on the remaining language tests. Subject 20 was adequately able to explain absurd sentences and syntactically and lexically ambiguous sentences.

Examination of subject 20's receptive language skills revealed relatively mild auditory comprehension deficits on both the Token Test of the NCCEA and the WST.

Case report 8 (Subject 41)

Subject 41, a 41-year-old female with 10 years of education reported a history of sensory problems with her right arm and leg since the age of 36. At the age of 39 years she was admitted to hospital after deterioration of her physical status resulted in an inability to talk. The diagnosis of RR MS was confirmed at that time by MRI scan. Neurological examination revealed reduced tone of the upper limbs with slight weakness of the left arm and hand. Reflexes were bilaterally brisk and ataxic on the left. Reduced power was also identified in both lower limbs with left sided ataxia, bilaterally brisk reflexes and upgoing plantar reflexes. The subject was wheelchair bound and incontinent of urine and faeces. Sensory loss was identified for light touch and vibration. Fundal examination revealed a pale left optic disc, an afferent defect in the left eye and reduced vision in the right eye. Some nystagmus on upward and downward gaze and bilateral intranuclear ophthalmoplegia with left palsy of the abducens nerve was identified. She presented with partial right lower motor neurone facial nerve palsy resulting in a mild dysarthria. Hospitalization and treatment with methylprednisone at this time improved some of her neurological signs and symptoms.

A repeat MRI scan two years later revealed innumerable foci of high signal intensities scattered throughout the white matter of each centrum semiovale, reported to be typical of MS (see Figure 9.3). Several of the plaques seen on MRI demonstrated enhancement after gadolinium infusion. There were also several plaques in the midbrain, pons, rostral medulla and left middle cerebellar peduncle. The size of the ventricles and sulci were slightly large for the subject's age but there was no mass effect above or below the tentorium. The radiologist concluded that the MRI reflected typical features of MS affecting the deep white matter of both hemispheres with several enhancing and several non-enhancing plaques indicating different stages of evolution. Borderline abnormality was identified in the optic chiasm consistent with an enlarged right side of the chiasm and minimal enhancement was concluded to be consistent with optic neuritis.

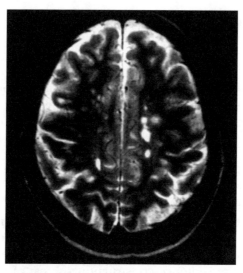

Figure 9.3 A magnetic resonance image revealing innumerable foci of high signal intensities scattered throughout the white matter of each centrum semiovale, reported to be typical of multiple sclerosis (T_2 weighted image with spin echo sequence TE/TR = 80/2143) for multiple sclerosis subject 41

At the time of language assessment the subject presented with perceptibly normal speech; however, she reported some slurring and slowing of her speech when fatigued. Subject 41 presented with intact abilities when visual naming, tactile naming with the right hand and describing the use of simple objects on the NCCEA. Her sentence repetition, digit repetition, digit reversal, reading, writing and articulation skills were all within normal limits.

The subject's completion of high-level measures of expressive and receptive linguistic ability revealed that her language was compromised on selected tasks. Word-finding difficulties were identified on lexical accessing tasks such as the BNT and the word fluency subtest of the NCCEA, which were relatively more complex than the visual naming subtest of the NCCEA. Left-handed tactile naming deficits on the NCCEA were also recorded. Subject 41's performance on the task requiring her to access synonyms and antonyms, however, was within normal limits relative to the control group.

Subject 41 demonstrated some difficulties with verbal explanation tasks on TWT and the TLC. She provided inadequate responses when explaining absurd sentences and the meanings of words. One of the inadequate explanations she provided for task C of TWT was the response 'He didn't actually neglect it' for the absurd sentence 'He neglected the puppy because he loved it so much' where she failed to relate accurately the meaning of the sentence in order to explain its absurd nature.

For some of the items on the making associations task, the subject selected the incorrect item from the group, which did not belong to the category, and also provided an inaccurate reason for her choice. Her interpretations of the metaphors in the TLC were also inadequate but she was able to select a matching metaphor from a choice of four. For instance, in the situation 'Two students talking about a teacher' the interpretation she provided for the expression 'It's hard to zero in on his ideas' was 'His ideas are different to what they're used to.' In this example, she did not express the notion that the speaker does not make himself clear but she did, however, correctly select the matching meaning which was 'His ideas do not come through.'

Subject 41 was able to provide at least one meaning for most of the ambiguous sentences in the TLC. The Making Inferences subtest revealed that she had difficulties selecting a single accurate conclusion for some of the stories presented. Although subject 41 performed within normal limits on the sentence construction subtest of the NCCEA, she made a number of errors recreating sentences on the TLC. Examination of her responses revealed that she produced semantically and syntactically inaccurate and, in some cases, incomplete sentences. The intact sentences that were produced, however, incorporated all three of the lexical items specified in the subtest.

Subject 41 performed well below average on the Token Test of the NCCEA which was suggestive of poor auditory comprehension abilities. Her performance, however, on the WST was only indicative of mild receptive language difficulties.

Case reports – Language subgroup 4 (near normal language abilities)

Case report 9 (Subject 21)

Subject 21 was a 41-year-old male with 10 years of education who reported that he had experienced his first symptoms of MS at the age of 26 years. Symptoms included right-sided weakness, visual disturbances and an inability to talk. He reported gradual deterioration of his physical status whereby he eventually became wheelchair dependent at the age of 40 years. An MRI scan taken at that time confirmed the diagnosis of CP MS. Scanning of the cervical spine excluded disc pathology, as the craniocervical junction and the cervical cord had a normal appearance. In addition, there was no evidence of spinal stenosis. An MRI scan of the cranium, however, revealed some high frequency areas in the periventricular regions particularly in the centrum semiovale on the left side (see Figure 9.4). There was also involvement of the internal capsule on

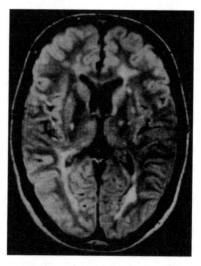

Figure 9.4 A magnetic resonance image showing some high frequency areas in the periventricular regions including the internal capsule on both sides with no evidence of mass effect (T_2 weighted image with spin echo sequence TE/TR = 20/2500) for multiple sclerosis subject 21

both sides and in the splenium of the corpus callosum with no evidence of mass effect. The findings were reportedly consistent with the demyelinating process of MS.

At the time of language assessment, subject 21 had perceptibly normal speech but he reported short-term memory problems. He said he stumbled over words at times and found he sometimes 'lost the thread' of the conversation. Subject 21 presented with intact visual and tactile naming for simple objects on the NCCEA. He was able to describe the use of objects and attained scores within normal limits relative to an adult reference population on tasks assessing sentence repetition, digit repetition, digit reversal, reading, writing and articulation.

Examination of subject 21's high-level expressive and receptive language abilities revealed minimal evidence of dysfunction. Word-finding skills were largely unimpaired as indicated by normal naming on the BNT and an intact ability to access synonyms and antonyms on TWT. The test of word fluency, however, revealed a marginally reduced score.

Varying levels of performance were exhibited by subject 21 on the verbal explanation tasks. He demonstrated an intact ability to explain absurd sentences and make reasonable inferences following presentation of a story. His definitions for some of the test words, however, were inadequate as were his interpretations for a number of the metaphorical expressions in the TLC. Although he had problems explaining some of the metaphors, he was able to select the correct matching meaning from a choice of four. The subject exhibited mild deficits when interpreting both syntactically and lexically ambiguous sentences. Examination of his responses revealed that he could identify a single meaning for most of the ambiguous items.

The finding of intact sentence construction abilities, identified on the simple task of the NCCEA, was not supported by the subject's performance on the recreating sentences subtest of the TLC. On the TLC task, subject 21 tended to produce deviant sentences in an attempt to incorporate the combination of three relatively more complex words into his response. For example, for the picture 'About moving' using the words 'difficult', 'nonetheless' and 'now' he produced the poorly constructed sentence 'It might be difficult to move nonetheless now.' His performance was also mildly impaired on TWT task requiring him to make associations. On some of the items, he selected the inappropriate word which did not belong to the category of the other three words and also provided insufficient reasons for the choice of the word. For instance, he selected the incorrect word 'rectangle' from a choice of lexical items 'wheel', 'rectangle', 'circle' and 'square' and gave the insufficient explanation 'it's not round'.

Although the presence of mild expressive language difficulties were identified in the assessments, subject 21's receptive language was found to be largely intact. Although his score on the Token Test of the NCCEA suggested mildly impaired auditory comprehension abilities, he attained a maximum score on the WST reflecting competent logico-grammatical processing skills.

Case report 10 (Subject 40)

Subject 40, a 25-year-old female with 10 years of education was first admitted to hospital at age 23 years with a history of increasing ataxia and a one week history of worsening ataxia, confusion, nausea and vomiting. She had experienced many vague neurological signs including a global decrease in higher functions presenting with reduced attention and concentration, constructional apraxia and poor verbal fluency, abstraction, calculation, writing skills and receptive language functions. Initial neurological examination revealed her to be grossly ataxic with limb ataxia worse on the left side. She had increased tone in her legs, bilateral hyperreflexia and bilateral extensor plantar responses. She experienced parasthesia in both upper limbs. A visual examination revealed that her fundi were normal but that her eye movements were jerky with pursuit and she had hypometric saccades. The subject presented with a brisk jaw jerk and dysarthria. Cerebrospinal examination revealed a pleocytosis of 27, a mildly elevated protein of 0.57 but negative india ink and cryptococcal antigen. Her human immunodeficiency virus and syphilis serologies were negative. An EEG revealed diffuse slow wave activity. Two CT scans performed and interpreted by a qualified radiologist showed diffuse periventricular low attenuation plus discrete areas of low attenuation in the deep white matter.

An MRI scan revealed multiple intra-cranial lesions (see Figure 9.5). They presented as multiple irregular round, mostly focal areas of increased signal intensity distributed throughout the deep white matter of both the cerebellar and cerebral hemispheres. They were notable in the right cerebellar hemispheres, both cerebellar peduncles, in the right basal ganglia, in the right side genu of the corpus callosum, and extensively in the periventricular regions adjacent to and above the bodies of both lateral ventricles. Larger more confluent areas of increased signal intensity were seen in the deep white matter posterior to both ventricular trigones. None of these lesions appeared to exert a mass effect. The results of the MRI were found to be more in favour of lymphoma or gross demyelination than progressive multifocal leukoencephalopathy.

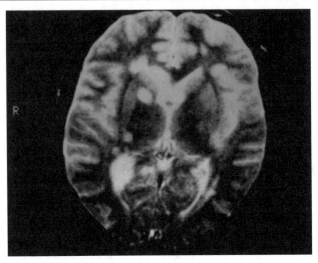

Figure 9.5 A magnetic resonance image revealing multiple irregular round, mostly focal areas of increased signal intensity distributed throughout the deep white matter of both cerebral hemispheres including the right basal ganglia (T_2 weighted image with spin echo sequence TE/TR = 85/3000) for multiple sclerosis subject 40

The clinical signs exhibited by the subject in combination with the neuroradiological findings, particularly multiple areas of discrete abnormal signals on the T_2 weighted images, were considered to be suggestive of a demyelinating disease consistent with a RR form of MS. Over the next few days her memory and attention difficulties slowly improved and she was discharged from hospital.

A neurological examination carried out just prior to the language assessment found that the subject presented with improved neurological signs and cognitive abilities. She had a wide-based ataxic gait with spasticity, bilateral cerebellar signs in the limbs (worse on the left side) and bilateral pyramidal signs with brisk reflexes and extensor plantar responses.

At the time of language assessment the subject presented with perceptibly normal speech; however, she reported that she often got her 'words tangled' making her speech hesitant on occasions. Intact visual naming, right-handed tactile naming, reading, writing and articulation abilities were indicated by subject 40's performance on the NCCEA. The subject also demonstrated the ability to describe the use of simple objects and repeat sentences. Difficulties, however, were experienced when she completed the digit repetition, digit reversal and left-handed tactile naming tasks.

Subject 40 performed similarly to the control group on many of the high-level language assessments. Preserved word-finding abilities were indicated by the subject's performance on the BNT and the synonym and antonym tasks of TWT. She attained scores only marginally below normal on the word fluency subtest of the NCCEA. In addition, the subject demonstrated an intact ability to make inferences, categorize objects and use verbal reasoning techniques. Some mild expressive language deficits were revealed when subject 40 provided inadequate explanations for three of the absurd sentences and poor scoring definitions for some of the lexical items on TWT. An example of an error she made on task E of TWT was the inadequate definition 'nice and cool' for the item 'air conditioner'.

Marginally low scores were attained by subject 40 when she explained syntactically and lexically ambiguous sentences and interpreted metaphors. The relatively low scores on these tasks, however, reflected erroneous responses on only a small number of the test items. The lowest score subject 40 achieved was on the recreating sentences subtest of the TLC. In this subtest, she used the three presented words to create her response but failed to include contextually related expressions of intent as indicated by the stimulus picture. On the simpler sentence construction task in the NCCEA, however, she was found to perform adequately without time constraints.

Subject 40 presented with intact auditory comprehension skills as indicated by relatively normal performance on the Token Test of the NCCEA and the WST.

Case report 11 (Subject 46)

Subject 46 was a 49-year-old female with 12 years of education who reported that she had experienced her first symptoms of MS at the age of 36 years when she kept falling over for no apparent reason. Her neurologist gave her a provisional diagnosis of MS. At the age of 47, she was admitted to hospital with a history of parasthesia. A neurological examination revealed bilaterally symmetrical hyperreflexia, bilateral extensor plantar responses (right greater than left) and mildly reduced vibration sense perception below the ankles. Although she complained of misty vision bilaterally, a visual examination revealed that her fundi were normal. Cerebrospinal examination revealed a mildly elevated protein level of 68g/L (63–80), but her syphilis serologies were non-reactive. The clinical findings were suggestive of a RR form of MS.

An MRI scan taken five months later confirmed the presence of a demyelinating disease and the diagnosis of MS. The scan revealed several small areas of increased signal intensity within the left cerebellar peduncle, the periventricular regions, the right centrum semiovale and the deep parietal white matter (see Figure 9.6). Neurological examination performed at the same time revealed persistent parasthesia and weakness in her lower limbs, reduced plantar reflexes, a positive Romberg's sign, impaired co-ordination and sensory ataxia.

At the time of language testing the subject was in remission and independently mobile. Her speech was perceptibly normal but she reported word-finding difficulties and the production of spoonerisms, particularly when reading aloud. Subject 46 was able to visually name, tactually name and describe the use of simple objects on the NCCEA. Her abilities to repeat sentences, repeat and reverse sequences of digits, reverse digits, read, write and articulate were all within normal limits. Intact word-finding skills were demonstrated on the BNT, word fluency task of the NCCEA, and tasks B and D on TWT requiring the subject to retrieve synonyms and antonyms.

Mildly impaired expressive and receptive language skills were evident, however, when subject 46 completed the remaining high-level language assessments. Her abilities to define words and explain three of the absurd sentences in TWT were suggestive of mild impairment relative to the control group. For example, on task E, for the item 'flash-light' subject 46 provided the inadequate definition 'a light', failing to include the critical element that the item is portable. In addition, scores just below the normal range were attained by subject 46 when she made inferences, explained ambiguous sentences and recreated sentences. Examination of her responses, however, revealed that she was able to provide at least one correct meaning for each of the syntactically or

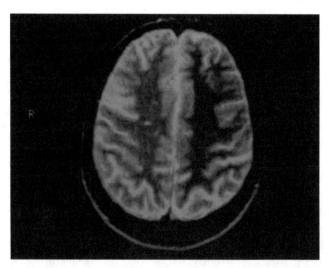

Figure 9.6 A magnetic resonance image showing several small areas of increased signal intensity in the right centrum semiovale (T_2 weighted image with spin echo sequence TE/TR = 85/3000) for multiple sclerosis subject 46

lexically ambiguous sentences. Although subject 46 performed well on the sentence construction task of the NCCEA, three of her sentences on the TLC recreating sentences subtest contained minor deviations. She exhibited a competent ability, however, to include all three words and take into account situational contexts when constructing her responses. Subject 46 presented with unimpaired verbal explanation skills when required to categorize items according to class name and associated semantic features, and then verbalize a reason the selected item did not belong to the category. She also was able to explain adequately the metaphors included in the TLC and able to select a matching metaphor for the item from a selection of four.

In comparison to the control group, subject 46 presented with auditory comprehension skills which were just below the normal range. Examination of the raw scores attained by the subject on both the Token Test of the NCCEA and the WST, however, did not appear to reflect a clinically relevant difference.

Neuroanatomical substrate of language variability in multiple sclerosis

Diverse performances on the language tasks, neurological histories, MS signs and symptoms and so on, as reported for each case in this chapter, are not surprising considering that MS is a neurological disorder which can affect the myelin sheath in any part of the central nervous system (CNS) (Beatty et al., 1990). Indeed, researchers have outlined the heterogeneous nature of the MS population in terms of the subjects' physical symptoms and disease course (Beatty et al., 1990), neuropsychological deficits (Bennett, 1989; Minden et al., 1990; Schiffer and Caine, 1991; Tolosa and Alvarez, 1992), neuroradiological pathology (Kirshner et al., 1985; Barnes et al., 1991) and the history of MS lesions (Nesbit et al., 1991).

Although the MS subjects described above presented with varied language deficits, the majority of the cases demonstrated expressive language deficits when compared with adult reference populations. Eight of the subjects exhibited impaired naming skills (e.g. subjects 4, 11, 12, 16, 20, 24, 26, 41) and nine subjects presented with reduced word fluency abilities (e.g. 4, 12, 16, 20, 21, 24, 26, 40, 41). As reported by Lethlean and Murdoch (1994a), the difficulties that MS subjects experience on confrontation naming tasks appear to arise from a lexical accessing deficit and/or compromised visual acuity. Verbal fluency deficits have been reported by a number of researchers as a common neuropsychological finding in MS which has been closely related to compromised cognitive processing (Margolin et al., 1990). According to

Margolin et al. (1990), the interpretation of an individual's performance on confrontation naming tasks and letter category verbal fluency tasks relies on examination of the cognitive processes required to perform them. Performance on semantic retrieval tasks has been correlated with other tasks involving primary attention, language and memory (Obler et al., 1986). In addition, it has been suggested that MS subjects' difficulty on verbal fluency tasks may be attributed to their inability to process information quickly (Beatty et al., 1988; Beatty, Monson and Goodkin, 1989; Beatty and Monson, 1990) independent of motor involvement (Rao, St. Aubin-Faubert et al., 1989). Beatty and Monson (1990) suggested that although MS subjects appear to have an intact semantic memory structure, they have difficulty with verbal fluency tasks which require an active and systematic search of semantic memory.

Obler et al. (1986) have reported that, in order to complete a word fluency task, subjects require the ability to sustain their attention to a category, search their memory, employ lexical retrieval strategies and translate a retrieved concept to an appropriate label. Attentional deficits (often featuring as generalized fatigue) and compromised memory abilities are commonly reported cognitive problems in people with MS (Rao, 1986). In fact, examination of subject 20's and 26's neuropsychological assessment results revealed features of reduced attention (subject 20) and memory deficits (subjects 26 and 20) associated with poor word fluency skills.

Word fluency deficits have been attributed to damage in the left frontal lobe (Goodglass and Kaplan, 1979; Jouandet and Gazzaniga, 1979). Indeed, subject 26's poor word fluency and uniformly low scores on the reported cognitive assessments were attributed by a neuropsychologist to a frontal type dyspraxia. Further, the MS cases described above exhibited multiple areas of increased signal intensity throughout the deep white matter on MRI which may have interfered with frontal cortico-subcortical connections (e.g. subjects 24, 26 and 41). In the absence of normal subcortical input to the frontal lobe, it is suggested that demyelination in the CNS associated with MS may have contributed to the MS subjects' compromised word fluency skills.

Researchers have suggested that corpus callosum demyelination, identified on MRI, provides the best explanation for cognitive deficits in the MS population (Gean-Marton et al., 1991). Corpus callosum atrophy identified on MRI has been considered a useful predictor of mental processing speed (e.g. verbal fluency) and rapid problem-solving ability, which depend on precisely timed interhemispheric communication (Rao, Bernardin et al., 1989; Pozzilli, Bastianello et al., 1991). Subject 21 presented with pockets of high-level language deficits which may have been attributed to the presence of high-frequency areas in the splenium of the corpus callosum on his MRI scan. His confrontation naming abilities were intact but his performance on the word fluency task, requiring sustained attention, mental processing speed and so on, was marginally impaired. He had some difficulties defining words, explaining metaphors and constructing sentences, whereas his receptive high-level language functions were intact.

Some of the MS subjects presenting with global high-level language deficits including expressive and receptive difficulties (e.g. subjects 24 and 26) and selective high-level language deficits (e.g. subjects 20 and 41), were found to exhibit high signal intensities in the white matter on MRI. Focal high signal intensity regions adjacent to the ventricles have been reported as a common finding in MS (Kirshner et al., 1985; Haughton et al., 1992) and, according to Haughton et al. (1992), these foci correspond to plaques of demyelination. In the literature, white matter lesions have been considered as a critical prerequisite to language dysfunction in subjects who have suffered a subcortical cerebrovascular accident (CVA) (Alexander et al., 1987). It has become widely accepted that language processing requires the integrity of cortical and subcortical structures and their pathways. Hart et al. (1985) have suggested that information processing by MS subjects depends on the integrity of their subcortical structures and white matter tracts. Subjects with extensive periventricular demyelination have been found to demonstrate an inferior performance on concept formation, non-verbal reasoning and verbal memory (Anzola et al., 1990). Among the MS cases described above, it is speculated that demyelination in cortico-subcortical and cortico-cortical pathways may have contributed to the MS subjects' poor performances on the high-level language tasks, which required extensive information processing. For example, subject 41's MRI scan exhibited innumerable foci of high signal intensity scattered throughout the deep white matter of both hemispheres, potentially interfering with normal subcortico-cortical communication. Her performance on the language tests, four months after MRI, revealed word-finding difficulties on the BNT and the word fluency task of the NCCEA, poor verbal explanations, inadequate interpretations of figurative language and impaired sentence construction abilities on subtests of TWT and the TLC, and mild auditory comprehension deficits on the NCCEA and the WST. Hence, subject 41's impaired high-level language abilities were apparent in the absence of cortical lesions identified on MRI.

Examination of the MS subjects' expressive naming and high-level language deficits documented in the cases described above may be explained, in part, using Wallesch and Papagno's (1988) subcortical model of language processing. Wallesch and Papagno (1988) have suggested that the basal ganglia and the thalamus play a role in language processing and that interruption of cortico-striato-pallido-thalamo-cortical loops leads to impaired language abilities. It is proposed that the consistent feature of impaired naming found in 8 of the 11 MS subjects described in this chapter may be attributed to an interrupted thalamic gating mechanism (Wallesch and Papagno, 1988). Potential cortico-subcortical disconnection in the MS group (White, 1990), interfering with ventral thalamic projections on the frontal language area, may lead to closure of the thalamic gates and the release of poorly monitored responses during confrontation naming. Although naming deficits following subcortical lesions have been explained in terms of an inaccurate thalamic gating mechanism, Wallesch and Papagno (1988) have suggested that in subjects with chronic diseases of the subcortical system (e.g. Parkinson's disease) naming abilities may remain largely undisturbed. Indeed, in the present chapter, the MS subjects 21, 40 and 46 all presented with preserved naming abilities. According to Wallesch and Papagno (1988), in a confrontation naming task, a limited number of responses can be formulated by the parallel modules in order to fit the criteria specified by the cortex. If all the parallel modules come up with the same response, even with a disturbed thalamic gating mechanism in some cases, there is no competition and the correct name will be produced.

The MS subjects' word fluency and verbal explanation deficits and relatively intact repetition abilities may be explained in terms of Wallesch and Papagno's (1988) degrees of freedom. Generation of names on word fluency tasks and lexical content in the spontaneous production of speech are divergent skills which allow many degrees of freedom. That is, in divergent language production, many more responses can be generated that fit the criteria proposed by the cortex, which in turn, require integration and selection by the subcortical structures. For example on TWT, there are many more possible responses a subject can produce when asked for a definition of a word (e.g. define the word 'stadium') in comparison to a task requiring fewer degrees of freedom such as the production of a synonym where the semantic field is already accessed (e.g. provide a synonym for the word 'repair'). Indeed, the subjects tended to perform more poorly when defining some words in comparison to their results on the synonym and antonym subtests (e.g. subjects 11 and 41). For example, subject 41 provided a number of inadequate definitions (e.g. 'It wouldn't be a bandstand would it?' for the word 'stadium'). Her ability to access synonyms and antonyms, however, was similar to the control group. Similarly, sentence repetition is a task which has small degrees of freedom, requires minimal integration by the basal ganglia, and is often undisturbed following compromised subcortical functioning (Wallesch and Papagno, 1988). It is suggested that most of the MS subjects' intact repetition of the content of the sentences while maintaining their surface structure is consistent with Wallesch and Papagno's (1988) model.

Interpretation of the metaphorical expressions on the TLC and explanation of absurdities on TWT, which are both divergent tasks with large degrees of freedom, require intact spontaneous language production abilities. It is speculated that the large degrees of freedom characterizing these tasks may explain the MS subjects' inadequate explanations of some of the metaphors (e.g. subjects 4, 12, 16, 20, 21 and 41) and absurd sentences (e.g. subjects 4, 12, 16, 24, 26 and 41). Although they had difficulty explaining the metaphors, once degrees of freedom were restricted and a multiple choice task was provided, some of the subjects were able to select the appropriate matching metaphor from a choice of four alternatives (e.g. subjects 12, 20, 21 and 41).

A number of the MS subjects were able to produce at least one meaning for the ambiguous sentences on the TLC but failed to provide a second meaning for some of the lexical items (e.g. subjects 11, 21 and 41). Wallesch and Papagno's (1988) model appears to explain the subjects' difficulties with this TLC subtest in terms of interruption to only some of the modular pathways in the subcortical system. The parallel modules originating in the cortex form cortico-striato-pallido-thalamo-cortical loops which, when uninterrupted, may provide all the possible meanings of the ambiguous sentences. If all the pathways are interrupted, however, the subject may produce an inaccurate meaning for the ambiguous sentence or fail to produce a response. If information in only one of the parallel modules is uninterrupted and allowed to complete the circuit, the production of only one meaning may result. For example, when subject 41 interpreted the sentence 'I saw the girl take his picture', the globus pallidus, under the influence of the striatum, appeared to accurately control and modulate by inhibiting the gating mechanism of the thalamus via pallido-thalamic fibres. Inhibition of the thalamus closed the thalamic gate which reduced the inhibition of the frontal cortex and led to the production of the modules containing the similar responses 'I saw the girl take his picture with a camera' and 'she could have taken a photo'. Her inability to provide a correct alternative meaning (i.e. 'I saw the girl take his picture from him'), however, may have been attributed to interrupted parallel cortico-subcortical modules.

Wallesch and Papagno (1988) have proposed that the basal ganglia act to integrate information. It is suggested that compromised white matter fibres connecting the cortical and subcortical structures may have contributed to the MS subjects' poor performance on the sentence construction subtest of the TLC. Examination of their responses revealed inadequately structured, poorly monitored sentences in an attempt to include the three specified words and the pragmatic context in the sentences. It is speculated that the MS subjects' subcortical structures failed to participate optimally in the selection of words as meaningful, conceptually adequate units (Cappa and Vignolo, 1979). For example, using the picture 'In the cafeteria' and the words 'pie', 'either' and 'have', subject 41 produced the semantically and syntactically inaccurate sentence 'The lady went to the pie shop but it was such a big decision as to whether have either pie (pause) to decide she's have to get two of them'.

A number of MS subjects also demonstrated difficulties on the categorization task of TWT, which required them to categorize four items, select the item which did not belong to the group and provide a reason for their choice (e.g. subjects 16, 20, 26, 41 and 21). Goodglass and Kaplan (1979) proposed that a reduced ability to deal with relationships between objects and their properties reflects impaired conceptual thinking and interruption to normal brain functioning. Once again, it is speculated that the MS subjects' failure to adequately perform this TWT verbal explanation task may have been attributed to compromised white matter pathways interfering with the critical input of the subcortical structures.

Overall, expressive high-level language deficits identified in the profiles of the present MS cases may be explained by compromised attentional and self monitoring functions of the subcortical structures which influence the frontal lobes (Wallesch and Papagno, 1988). It has already been suggested that inaccurate thalamic gating mechanisms and poor self-monitoring may lead to the MS subjects' production of naming errors on confrontation naming tasks. In addition, it is proposed that the subjects' relatively poor performances on the cognitive/linguistic tasks of the TLC may have been attributed, in part, to incompetent self-monitoring mechanisms. While the MS subjects appeared to understand the task requirements at the time of testing, they seemed to have difficulty using feedback to compare the responses they produced with the given test requirements. Some of the MS subjects did not comment on the inappropriate responses which they produced for some of the linguistic tasks, whereas the control subjects expressed difficulty and dissatisfaction with a task they felt had not been adequately completed. This was particularly apparent when the MS subjects attempted the sentence construction subtest of the TLC. On many items they produced inaccurate or ungrammatical sentences in an attempt to include the three required words but failed to monitor that the sentences were incorrect. For example, when asked to construct a sentence using the words 'difficult', 'now' and 'nonetheless' in the context of 'moving house', subject 12 produced the ungrammatical sentence 'Nonetheless the last furniture had to go now being difficult'.

Alternatively, the MS subjects failed to monitor their responses by not complying with the instructions to include all three words in one sentence. Some of their erroneous responses only included two of the specified words in a recreated sentence, whereas other inadequate productions were comprised of two grammatical sentences using the three words. In these cases, the subjects failed to monitor their responses and compare them with the task requirements. For example, when required to create a sentence using the words 'before', 'rather' and 'after' in response to the picture 'At the movie theatre', subject 4 produced the sentence 'Before we go to the movies I'd rather have something to eat. After the movie's finished I'll have a cup of coffee'. In contrast, the control subjects carefully monitored their responses, expressed dissatisfaction and revised their answers if they created an ungrammatical sentence or failed to include all three words. In completing the tasks, it seems that the MS subjects lost the regulating influence on their linguistic responses as a result of interruptions to subcortical feedback neural systems. However, further research is required to explore this suggestion.

Wiig and Secord (1985) have suggested that the tasks on the TLC require intact problem-solving and planning abilities. It has been proposed that an inability to complete the stages of processing required for problem-solving tasks, including a higher-order feedback stage, is indicative of impaired frontal lobe functioning (Nadeau, 1991). Indeed, the MS subjects exhibited a number of cognitive/linguistic deficits which have been reported to occur in neurologically impaired individuals with primarily frontal lobe deficits (e.g. poor word fluency, planning, self monitoring and problem-solving skills) (Jouandet and Gazzaniga, 1979). Swirsky-Sacchetti et al. (1992) have found that left frontal lobe involvement in MS best predicted impaired abstract problem-solving, memory and word fluency. Forebrain lesion load has been closely related to measures of cognitive and memory impairment (Rao, Leo et al., 1989). Hence, it is possible that the linguistic deficits associated with subcortical white matter impairment identified in the present MS group may be attributed to an indirect effect on the cortical structures important for language processing (e.g. frontal lobe).

Language deficits associated with a CVA involving the subcortical structures and cortico-subcortical pathways may be attributed to indirect effects on the cortex (Metter et al., 1988; Vallar et al., 1988). Changes in cortical function may reflect the loss of important information from the subcortical structures due to diaschisis (Metter, 1987). Impaired cortical metabolism and blood flow that occur following lesions of the thalamus, internal capsule and basal ganglia, have provided further evidence that cortico-subcortical connections are critical for language performance (Metter et al., 1988; Vallar et al., 1988). Similarly, cortico-subcortical disconnection has been proposed as the most likely cause of cognitive dysfunction in MS where reduced metabolism in the grey matter may reflect cortical suppression secondary to disconnection from subcortical structures (Brooks et al., 1984; Pozzilli et al., 1993; Pugnetti et al., 1993). Indeed, disconnection effects may have contributed to the high-level language deficits identified in the language profiles of the MS subjects described above. It seems that diffuse white matter demyelination or multiple focal lesions in MS which potentially compromise cortico-subcortical connections may have a similar disconnection effect as reported to occur in focal subcortical cerebrovascular accidents involving the white matter. Whether or not the subcortical structures have a direct and/or an indirect role in language processing, there is a close functional relationship between the frontal lobe and the subcortical structures in linguistic and cognitive processing (Alexander et al., 1986). This functional relationship may explain similar cognitive/ linguistic deficits which occur following lesions in different areas of the frontal lobe system (Cummings and Benson, 1988). Further studies are required to determine the potential distance effects of inflammation and oedema of MS white matter lesions and chronic focal MS lesions on the cortical and subcortical structures. In addition, further research is required to elucidate the effect of fluctuating lesions on language task performance and to consider the influence of MS pathology producing a retardation rather than a cessation of neural transmission (Bennett, 1989), on linguistic abilities.

Although comments have been made in the present discussion concerning the possible neuroanatomical basis for the MS subjects' language deficits, it is recognized that the lesions on the MRI scans which have been reported in this chapter are likely to have changed over time. Serial studies of MS subjects with a RR disease course have revealed considerable changes on MRI scans within a four week period (Isaac et al., 1988; Capra et al., 1992; Rudick, 1992). The MRI scans for the MS subjects described above were taken months and, in some cases, years both before and after the language tasks were administered, so it is likely that the number, location and activity of lesion sites may have changed. For example, subject 40's MRI scan was taken when she had an acute relapse of MS and, according to her medical records, concurrently exhibited considerably impaired cognitive and language abilities. Evaluation of subject 40's high-level language abilities in the present study, after her MS had gone into remission, however, revealed largely unimpaired linguistic functions.

Some studies of MS have demonstrated a strong relationship between plaque burden in the cerebrum on MRI and neuropsychological performance (Anzola et al., 1990; Baumhefner et al., 1990; Huber et al., 1992), whereas others have not identified a significant correlation (Litvan et al., 1988; Feinstein et al., 1993). Researchers have suggested that pathological events in MS are more frequent and widespread than is evidenced by clinical signs and symptoms (Capra et al., 1992; Rudick, 1992; Thompson et al., 1992). Consequently, subjects may present with clinically silent lesions (Thompson et al., 1990; Feinstein et al., 1993). Kirshner et al. (1985) proposed that location of lesions may be more important than the number of lesions on MRI. In contrast, other researchers state that not only the site of the MS lesions but also their nature and activity (Thompson et al., 1990) and the efficiency of the recovery mechanisms in the damaged nerve fibres after remissions of the disease (McDonald, 1986) need to be considered. Despite small areas of increased signal intensity in the left cerebellar peduncle, the periventricular regions right centrum semiovale and deep parietal white matter, subject 46 was found to present with largely intact high-level language abilities. In this case, the location, size and activity of the white matter lesions apparent on MRI may not have acted to interfere with normal cortical and subcortical communication. Wallesch and Papagno (1988) have emphasized the parallel nature of the system in their model of language processing to account for those subjects presenting with interrupted subcortical input and no significant language deficit (e.g. subjects 40 and 46). They suggest that the subcortical nuclei are part of a functional system (e.g. frontal lobe system) where there are numerous projections upon the frontal language areas from other areas of the system (e.g. cortico-cortical links) and bypasses (e.g. bidirectional cortico-thalamo links) which allow plasticity of the system and functional reorganization. Similarly, recovery of cognitive deficits in individuals with a RR course of MS has been attributed to the inflammatory process subsiding and/or the role of plasticity of the brain (Pugnetti et al., 1993).

Examination of two of the globally language impaired subjects' neuroradiological CT and MRI reports revealed the presence of generalized atrophy in the cerebrum (i.e. subjects 20 and 24). In addition, the CT scan revealed that subject 24 had multiple areas of increased signal in the absence of focal lesions and subject 20's MRI scan revealed multiple focal areas of increased signal intensity throughout the periventricular white matter. The presence of cortical atrophy as well as deep subcortical white matter impairment, evident on subject 20's and subject 24's neuroradiological assessments, may explain, at least in part, their global expressive and receptive high-level language deficits.

Subjects with subcortical vascular lesions, the group on which Wallesch and Papagno's (1988) model was developed, tend to present with more isolated focal lesion sites compared with the present MS subjects' diffuse subcortical white matter lesions. Although some of the MS subjects' language deficits have been explained using Wallesch and Papagno's (1988) model, it is suggested that the different nature of the MS lesions influencing the pathways connecting both the cortico-subcortical and cortico-cortical pathways, complicated by the presence of cognitive deficits, needs to be addressed. Given the diffuse and variable involvement of the white matter tracts in MS, it is difficult to make precise statements concerning the neuroanatomical substrate that leads to high-level language deficits in this population. It seems that conclusions concerning the neuroanatomical basis for the MS subjects' language difficulties can only be made with further studies including neuroradiological investigations with measures of functional subcortical and cortical activity (e.g. metabolic studies), neuropsychological measures, and high-level language assessments.

Clinical implications of variable language performance in multiple sclerosis

The case reports presented in the present chapter demonstrate that the diagnosis of MS does not necessarily indicate that an individual will present with or develop high-level language deficits. Awareness of the MS subjects who present with mild language deficits, however, may be important for those clinicians involved in rehabilitation and re-employment programmes for persons with MS. For example, the presence of subtle language difficulties may impair an individual's ability to perform in the workplace (e.g. in reading and writing tasks, providing and comprehending complex instructions). Thus researchers and clinicians should endeavour to use a case-by-case method of assessing the language abilities of people with MS so that appropriate rehabilitation programmes tailored to the individual subject's needs can be developed and coping strategies recommended.

Chapter 10
Treatment of language disorders in multiple sclerosis

Fiona J Hinchliffe, Bruce E Murdoch and Deborah G Theodoros

Introduction

There has been an emergent acceptance that language and other cognitive deficits can occur in multiple sclerosis (MS) as a result of the sclerotic lesions involving white-matter tracts and subcortical structures of the brain (Rao et al., 1985; Filley et al., 1989; Mendez and Frey, 1992; Lethlean and Murdoch, 1994a, 1997; Arnott et al., 1997). Despite this recognition, the literature defining the nature of the language sequelae in MS and the impact of such disorders on functional communicative activity remains relatively limited. The previous three chapters have presented the nature of the linguistic disturbances found to occur in MS patients. The present chapter considers the impact of such linguistic impairment on communication skill and will expound the issues involved in treating language-based communicative deficits in MS.

Communication is fundamental to all levels of daily activity and effective communication is necessary for the maintenance of a positive quality of life and psychosocial well-being. Even the most subtle of communication impairments can seriously influence the success with which an individual achieves his or her occupational, personal and interpersonal goals. Because the onset of MS typically occurs in early adulthood and the disease course is most often protracted, many MS sufferers will develop and have to cope with communicative difficulties for the greater part of their adult lives. In addition, Farmakides and Boone (1960) observed that the ability for persons with MS to communicate effectively becomes increasingly important as they lose motor control and progressively become more physically dependent on others. Consideration by speech-language pathologists of remediation programmes that ameliorate the language disorders and resulting communicative impairment secondary to MS is, therefore, warranted.

Approaches to the rehabilitation of communication impairment in multiple sclerosis

It is now recognized that MS can result in cognitive (Bennett et al., 1991; Rao, 1996) and high-level language narrative disorders (Arnott et al., 1997; Lethlean and Murdoch, 1997) which affect the ability to achieve effective and efficient communication. Hence, patients with MS may encounter what has been termed 'cognitive-communication disorders'. These are disorders of communication which result from impairments in linguistic and metalinguistic skill as well as nonlinguistic cognitive functions such as perception, discrimination, organization, reasoning, attention, and memory (ASHA, 1987, 1990). The presence of such impairments may cause an inability to comprehend subtlety in language, integrate spoken or written information, draw conclusions or give coherence to narrative. These types of neurobehavioural sequelae in MS have been likened to those that occur following closed head injury (Bennett et al., 1991; Rao, 1996; Arnott et al., 1997). These findings highlight the need for rehabilitation specialists to consider the functional effects of deficits in neuronal transmission secondary to diffuse axonal injury or disease.

Rehabilitation of neurobehavioural disorders including cognitive-communication impairments may be restorative or compensatory (Gross and Schultz, 1986; Diller, 1987; Levin, 1990; Coelho et al., 1996; Mazaux and Richer, 1998). The restorative approach assumes that repetitive exercise of neuronal circuits will facilitate neuronal growth and hence improve function. Thus, it aims to restore cognitive function within the context of its premorbid organization. In contrast, the compensatory approach assumes certain functions cannot be restored and is, therefore, aimed at developing skills and strategies to circumvent impaired ability and achieve functional competence (Mazaux and Richer, 1998). It has been argued, however, that it is artificial to separate restoration from compensation within a rehabilitation programme and that both approaches should be utilized simultaneously (Coelho et al., 1996).

The rehabilitation of MS patients is a distinct process and can be distinguished from the rehabilitation processes applied to other forms of acquired neurological dysfunction for a number of reasons. First, MS is a degenerative disease resulting in a progressive deterioration in functional activity. This progression may be chronic and occur in steady increments or may follow a relapsing-remitting pattern where deterioration followed by temporary restoration or improvement of function may occur (Rao et al.,1985) (see Chapter 1). In some cases of MS, however, it is likely that following each relapsing episode the residual functional deficits have been measurably exacerbated, thus contributing to a gradual decline in function. Because of the progressive nature of the MS, the primary focus of rehabilitation is most often on teaching compensatory strategies. Such strategies aim to alleviate the present difficulties by maximizing functional abilities and provide a foundation for greater compensatory needs should the level of impairment increase (Bennett et al., 1991). In earlier stages of the disease, however, some degree of restorative intervention, targeting specific components of cognitive-linguistic processes, may be indicated.

The heterogeneous nature of the linguistic deficits and the disease variables in MS must be considered when developing rehabilitation programmes for MS patients. The previous chapter has revealed that a single profile cannot adequately describe the language problems that accompany MS. Some individuals present with minimal deficits on tests requiring higher-order linguistic function, while others encounter pervasive language difficulties encompassing convergent and divergent linguistic ability. In addition, because of the variability of the disease process, each individual with MS presents with a unique profile of physical disability which may influence the nature of the communicative environment encountered by the individual. Any rehabilitation programme needs to consider the environmental constraints and demands encountered by the individual concerned.

In recent times, the rehabilitation of adults with acquired cognitive-communication deficits has been tailored towards refined conceptualizations of patient outcomes. Present practices adopt ecological approaches to achieving the functional outcomes seen as fundamental to a positive quality of life for the individual (Frattali, 1998a, b; Mazaux and Richer, 1998). In providing a rehabilitation programme to alleviate the communication handicap experienced by an MS patient, the clinician should consider a 'lifestyle' therapy programme. Essentially such therapy aims to minimize impairment, maximize potential and monitor change within the context of the individual's functioning sensory modalities and communicative environment. Interventions need to be socially valid and should be directed toward individually meaningful real-world outcomes that promote personal and community linkages. Therapy should strive to anticipate possible communication breakdowns and provide facilities to solve everyday problems so that the individual can maintain adequate social adaptation.

In contemporary health care settings the emphasis on measuring outcomes and cost-benefit relationships of rehabilitation has become critical. The efficiency and efficacy of the treatment provided needs to be monitored and measuring the success of the outcome may be vital to ensure ongoing fiscal support of the rehabilitation programme. The desired outcomes are necessarily individually determined entities. It is important that the 'stakeholders' are involved in the planning and monitoring of outcomes (Rosenthal, 1995). Stakeholders are those who have a vested interest in the outcome of treatment and may include the person with MS, their family members, service providers, friends and work associates. In essence, the clinician should strive to provide therapy which is conducted efficiently and which effectively achieves desired outcomes that are socially meaningful for the individual concerned.

Outcome measurement is, therefore, integral to any intervention for language-based communication disorders in MS. The World Health Organization (WHO) (1980) has produced the most widely recognized conceptual framework for describing consequential aspects of illness, the International Classification of Impairments, Disabilities and Handicaps (ICIDH). This classification provides a framework by which to assess the consequential phenomena of an illness and systematically structure an intervention programme and measure its outcome. The WHO framework represents the sequelae of an illness on a continuum of impairment, disability and handicap. According to this framework, impairment refers to any abnormality of function at the organ level. Disability is the functional consequence of an impairment and refers to 'any restriction or lack of ability to perform an activity in the manner or within the range considered normal for a human being' (WHO, 1980, p. 143). Handicap is the disadvantage resulting from an impairment or disability 'that limits or prevents the fulfilment of a role that is normal (depending on age, sex, and social and cultural factors) for that individual' (WHO, 1980, p. 183). A handicap is, therefore, the social consequence of an impairment or disability, and is defined by the attitudes and responses of others. For example, according to the WHO framework (1980), the consequences of MS on communication could be represented on a continuum of deficits in auditory processing, word finding, attention, and verbal organization (impairments), reduced ability in social interaction or pragmatic communication (disability), and an inability to fulfil a normal life role involving physical independence and vocational or family status (handicap).

Development of a therapy programme for communication deficits in MS

In formulating a comprehensive, cost-effective and successful language and communication therapy programme for an MS patient, the clinician may consider a step-wise, multi-level approach which assesses and targets the consequences of the illness at the levels of impairment, disability and handicap. Table 10.1 uses the WHO typology to illustrate this approach to assessment and treatment. Such a programme involves the following component steps: identification of the linguistic impairment; identification of the communicative environment; identification of the cognitive-communication disability and handicap; establishment of the treatment goals; implementation of treatment and monitoring of treatment outcome.

There is no empirical evidence to substantiate the effectiveness of any intervention for cognitive-communication deficits in MS. The information presented here can, therefore, only offer some educated suggestions for therapy approaches and clinical interventions with MS patients. The following information borrows from intervention strategies that

Table 10.1 Structure of assessment, intervention and outcome measurement for cognitive-communication disorder in multiple sclerosis according to the World Health Organization (WHO) classification framework

	Impairment	Disability	Handicap
DEFINITION	Abnormality of structure or function at the organ level	Functional consequences of an impairment	Social consequences of an impairment or disability
EXAMPLES	Auditory processing deficit	Difficulty comprehending lengthy instructions	Unable to perform job Social isolation
ASSESSMENT	Standardized diagnostic measures	Tests of discourse and functional communication	Quality of life scales Handicap inventories
TREATMENT	Modality-specific or Component process exercises	Compensatory activity Functional skills training	Environmental manipulation
OUTCOME MEASURE	Standardized diagnostic measures Therapy outcome measures	Functional status measures Therapy outcome measures	Quality of life scales Therapy outcome measures

Source: Adapted from World Health Organization (1980)

have been applied to other populations, such as those with traumatic brain injury and right hemisphere brain damage, who typically encounter deficits in cognitive-communicative function.

Identification of linguistic impairment

The first step in any rehabilitation programme is comprehensive assessment. It has been emphasized here in earlier chapters that the assessment of language at the impairment level should go beyond tests of primary language function to include standardized assessments of higher-order linguistic skills. The assessment should aim to sample all modalities of language processing in a hierarchical manner and should include evaluation of auditory and reading comprehension, lexical selection and retrieval, verbal and written expression, verbal memory and learning, verbal integration and semantic organization, abstract language use such as comprehension of humour, proverbs and idiomatic expression, and ability to use language for problem-solving and reasoning (Hartley, 1995). Table 10.2 lists suggested standardized assessment batteries, which include tests of primary language function as well as those that have been found to be sensitive to deficits of higher-order linguistic and metalinguistic ability (Lethlean and Murdoch, 1997; Hinchliffe et al., 1998). The results from these assessments should allow the clinician to determine the linguistic skill of the individual and identify the linguistic-based underpinnings for any communicative disability which is present.

Table 10.2 Suggested assessments for language impairment in multiple sclerosis

	Component process	Suggested test/subtest
Primary Language Processes	Auditory Comprehension – word level	Boston Diagnostic Aphasia Examination (BDAE) (Goodglass and Kaplan, 1983) Western Aphasia Battery (WAB) (Kertesz, 1982)
	Auditory Comprehension- sentence level/ commands	BDAE (Goodglass and Kaplan, 1983) – Following Commands. WAB (Kertesz, 1982) – Auditory Comprehension Revised Token Test (McNeil and Prescott, 1978)
	Auditory Comprehension – paragraph level	BDAE (Goodglass and Kaplan, 1983) – Complex Ideational Material

Table 10.2 (contd)

	Component process	Suggested test/subtest
	Oral Expression – Naming	Boston Naming Test (Kaplan et al., 1983) WAB (Kertesz, 1982) – Object Naming BDAE (Goodglass and Kaplan, 1983) – Picture Naming; Responsive Naming
	Oral Expression – Verbal Fluency	BDAE (Goodglass and Kaplan, 1983) and WAB (Kertesz, 1982) – Animal Naming Neurosensory Centre Comprehensive Examination for Aphasia (NCCEA) (Spreen and Benton, 1969) – Word Fluency Controlled Oral Word Association Test (COWAT) (Benton and Hamsher, 1983)
	Oral Expression – Sentence generation	NCCEA (Spreen and Benton, 1969) – Sentence Construction
	Oral Expression – Picture Description	BDAE (Goodglass and Kaplan, 1983) – Cookie Theft WAB (Kertesz, 1982) – Spontaneous Speech Content and Fluency Scales
	Reading Comprehension – Word Level	BDAE (Goodglass and Kaplan, 1983) WAB (Kertesz, 1982)
	Reading Comprehension – Sentence to Paragraph Level	BDAE (Goodglass and Kaplan, 1983) WAB (Kertesz, 1982)
	Written Expression	BDAE (Goodglass and Kaplan, 1983) WAB (Kertesz, 1982)
Higher-Order Language Processes	Auditory Comprehension and Reasoning	Test of Language Competence – Extended (TLC-E) (Wiig and Secord, 1989) – Listening Comprehension Wiig-Semel Test of Linguistic Concepts (Wiig and Semel, 1974)

(contd)

Table 10.2 (contd)

Component process	Suggested test/subtest
Semantic Knowledge and Expressive Vocabulary	The Word Test – Revised (TWT-R) (Huisingh et al., 1990)
Comprehension of ambiguity	TLC-E – Ambiguous Sentences
Comprehension of inferred meaning	TLC-E – Listening Comprehension: Making Inferences Right Hemisphere Language Battery (RHLB) (Bryan, 1989) – Comprehension of Inferred Meaning
Comprehension of absurdities	TWT-R – Semantic Absurdities
Comprehension of Humour	RHLB – Appreciation of Humour
Comprehension of figurative and idiomatic expression	RHLB – Metaphor Picture Test, Written Metaphor Test TLC-E – Figurative Language
Verbal reasoning and problem solving	TWT-R – Semantic Absurdities TLC-E – Listening Comprehension; Ambiguous Sentences

Identification of the communication environment and communicative handicap

In order to determine the impact of linguistic impairment on the communicative participation of the MS individual, it is necessary to observe the unique communicative environment of that individual. The MS patient may be living independently and require skills to maintain function within the community, or may be living in a supportive family situation where assistance for daily activity is available but independent function is also required. Alternatively, the person with MS may be residing in an institutional facility, which provides different levels of assistance depending on the physical needs of the person. All situations will necessitate different levels and types of communicative interaction.

As well as the place of residence, the daily activities of the patient must be considered. For example, some people with MS will be in a work environment, or may have an active role in their community, or may regularly attend organized social functions. It is, therefore, neces- sary to identify what regular activities the patient is involved in, then establish the communicative demands of each one and the possible environmental supports available. With this knowledge, the degree to which the person encounters communication handicap can be determined and compensatory intervention can be planned.

An environmental needs assessment or ecological inventory, such as the one proposed by Hartley (1995), would provide the clinician with a systematic method for identifying the present and future communicative environments of the individual and the activities, roles and communicative partners within those environments. Another structured approach for determining how important certain everyday communication skills are to MS individuals is *The Communication Profile* (Payne, 1994). This assessment lists 26 everyday functional communicative skills and requires the individual to rate, on a five-point scale, the importance of these skills to them in their daily lives. For example, the respondent is asked to rate how important activities such as reading a prescription label or talking on the telephone to family are to them.

Identification of cognitive-communication disability

Once the linguistic impairments have been delineated and the communicative requirements established, the clinician may assess the degree to which the linguistic deficit impacts on the functional communicative ability of the MS patient. Cognitive-linguistic impairments, such as an inability to comprehend subtlety in language or integrate verbal information, may lead to a disability in pragmatic communication and eventual social isolation.

Assessment of communication disability involves the evaluation of how the MS speaker effectively plans and delivers or understands message content in different interactive contexts. Thus, it is necessary to examine the discourse and pragmatic skills of the individual. Such an assessment will entail observation and measurement of functional communicative activity, along with consultation with the MS patient and other 'stakeholders'. Table 10.3 lists some suggested standardized and non-standardized methods for assessing functional communicative ability in persons with diffuse neurological disorders. These methods include direct and indirect measurements of functional skill. Indirect methods involve interviews, surveys, self-reports, or ratings by familiar communicative partners. Direct methods entail quantitative measures of discourse comprehension and production, and observation and rating of communicative ability in clinical and/or natural environments (Hartley, 1995).

Through assessment of interactive and discourse skills the clinician can establish how the linguistic deficits may impede the ability of the MS individual to perform activities that constitute his/her routines and participate meaningfully in society. The clinician should discuss with, and where necessary explain to, the MS patient and other stakeholders the functional consequences of the language impairment. The MS patient needs to possess a metacognitive awareness about their communication ability in order to understand and participate in the design of treatment strategies.

Table 10.3 Suggested assessments for communication disability in multiple sclerosis

Instrument	Communication abilities assessed	Assessment method	Standardization
Pragmatic Protocol (Prutting and Kirchner, 1987)	30 parameters rating abilities in verbal, paralinguistic and nonverbal aspects of communication.	15 minutes of unstructured conversation. Dimensions rated as appropriate, inappropriate or no opportunity to observe.	Standardized on RBD, LBD, non-brain damaged elderly
Scale for rating conversational ability (Ehrlich and Sipes, 1985)	13 aspects of conversational abilities.	5-point scale	Non-standardized
Conversational rating scale (Ehrlich and Barry, 1989)	6 parameters assessing quality of spontaneous conversation: intelligibility; eye gaze; sentence formulation; coherence of narrative; topic; initiation of communication.	9-point scale	Non-standardized
Conversational Skills Rating Scale (CSRS; Spitzberg and Hurt, 1987)	25 specific aspects of communicative ability and 5 global parameters.	5-point scale	Non-standardized
Checklist of Listening Behaviours (Hartley, 1990)	Rates observations of 17 behaviours pertinent to listening.	5-point scale	Non-standardized

Table 10.3 (contd)

Instrument	Communication abilities assessed	Assessment method	Standardization
Analysis of Topic (Hartley, 1995)	Worksheet for analysing frequency of topic initiation, maintenance and disruption.	Tally frequency of utterances which signal topic initiation, topic maintenance and topic disruption.	Non-standardized
Analysis of Monologic Discourse (See Hartley, 1995 for a summary of quantitative measures)	Clinical elicitation and analysis of narrative, procedural, expository or persuasive discourse along the dimensions of sentential structure, productivity, information content, cohesion and coherence	Variable	Non-standardized
Discourse Comprehension Test (DCT; Brookshire and Nicholas, 1993)	Comprehension of stated and implied main ideas and details in narratives.	Yes/no questions	Standardized on 20 RBD adults
Functional Communication Profile (FCP; Sarno, 1969)	45 communicative behaviours.	9-point scale	Standardized
ASHA Functional Assessment of Communication Skills for Adults (Frattali et al., 1995)	43 items assessing social communication, communication of basic needs, reading, writing, number concepts, daily planning.	7-point scale of independence; 5-point scale of qualitative dimensions of communication.	Standardized

RBD = right-hemisphere brain damaged; LBD = left-hemisphere brain damaged

Establishing the goals of treatment

In consultation with the MS patient and other stakeholders, the clinician needs to establish a set of realistic, specific and structured goals of treatment that are objective and measurable. These goals will depend on the communicative demands, the available support, and the cognitive-linguistic limitations experienced by the MS person. In addition, therapy should be planned with a full understanding of what is important for the patient and the significant people in their lives. In this way, the therapy will be socially valid and meaningful for the individual and, therefore, most likely to be motivational and ultimately successful.

Intervention for cognitive-communication deficits associated with MS requires a multi-level and multi-method approach. Figure 10.1 provides an example of a treatment plan in which intervention goals are defined at the levels of impairment, disability, and handicap. The intervention applied to reach the defined goals can involve multiple treatment methods. The first level of goal formation involves defining the desired long-term global outcome. This holistic goal addresses, in functional terms, the overall expected outcome for the individual. In other words, it specifies the degree to which the existing handicap can be overcome and the amount of participation the person aims to experience. For example, the long-term outcome for an individual with minimal physical difficulties may be to maintain the ability to live and communicate with minimal assistance in his/her own home. The second level of goal formation is to identify the intermediate goals aimed at attaining the functional skills required to achieve the long-term goal. For example, one goal may be that the person will be able to instruct a home-help as to the daily procedures and needs of the household. Hartley (1995) has summarized an extensive list of functional communication goals across different life domains such as the home, community and work environments. The third level of goal formation identifies the short-term or immediate objectives of treatment. These goals may target the modality-specific or component process skills which are required to attain the intermediate goals and it is at this level that simultaneous use of multiple therapeutic methods may be applied. These methods are discussed more fully in the next section.

Implementing treatment

Once the goals of treatment have been established, rehabilitation for the cognitive-communication deficits can commence. Effective rehabilitation must be conducted in an environment which is positive, consistent and well organized, and where the performance expectations are clearly understood, measured and reinforced.

Communication Therapy Programme

Name:

Date:

Communication Environment:
Home:

Work:

Communication Partners:
Home:

Work:

Motor Speech:

Long-term goal:

Baseline Measure:

Vision:

Motor Control:

Suggested Intervention:

Outcome Measure:

Mobility:

Intermediate Goals	Baseline Measure	Suggested Intervention	Outcome Measure	Immediate Goals	Baseline Measure	Suggested Intervention	Outcome Measure

Treatment Schedule:

Maintenance Schedule:

Figure 10.1 Example of a communication therapy plan targeting levels of impairment, disability and handicap

In achieving therapy goals, use of an integrated approach to intervention, which incorporates four of the methods of cognitive-communicative intervention identified by Hartley (1995), would be optimal. These include component process retraining, environmental manipulation, compensatory strategy training, and functional skills training. As Figure 10.1 illustrates, different treatment approaches are used to target different levels of function and to achieve different levels of defined goals. Component process retraining can be used to target the immediate goals which aim to ameliorate the specific cognitive-linguistic impairments identified through standardized testing and which underpin the functional communication disorder. Component process retraining often utilizes hierarchically organized work-book type activities which target higher-level linguistic, metalinguistic, and pragmatic operations. For example, this intervention may include exercises which target word retrieval skills, auditory processing, reading comprehension, verbal organization, or pragmatic ability. Table 10.4 presents a list of linguistic impairments common in MS individuals and suggested component process retraining activities. A list of widely used clinical resources for component process activities for higher-order cognitive-communication deficits can be found in the Appendix.

Table 10.4 Suggested therapy exercises for common linguistic impairments in multiple sclerosis

Impairment	Suggested therapy activity
Lexical-Semantic Processing	
Difficulty with identifying word meanings Difficulty identifying salient semantic features Difficulty with semantic categorization	Identifying synonyms and antonyms; semantic choice questions; defining words by class; defining words by attribute; defining using negation; matching words with definitions; defining words; producing multiple definitions; identifying correct meanings of homonyms and homophones; naming semantic categories; identifying semantic features of categories and category members; naming category members

Table 10.4 (contd)

Comprehension of spoken instructions

Difficulty following instructions with multiple critical elements	Following instructions which increase in number of critical semantic elements

Comprehension of lengthy or complex auditory information

Difficulty detecting and remembering main ideas Difficulty making inferences and drawing conclusions Difficulty interpreting abstract ideas Difficulty recognizing incongruency Difficulty discriminating relevant versus irrelevant information Difficulty recognizing incongruency Difficulty resolving ambiguity	Summarizing tasks; story retelling; answering specific questions; deriving punch-lines; anticipating next episode; interpreting abstract expressions; defining abstract expressions; recognizing correct interpretations of proverbs and/or metaphorical statements; distinguishing fact from opinion in isolated statements and in connected argument; providing definitions for multiple-meaning words; identifying phrases with multiple meanings arising from surface- or deep- structure characteristics; using semantic, syntactic and pragmatic cues to accurately interpret embedded multiple-meaning sentences in narratives; produce non-literal meaning of words

Comprehension of complex written information

Difficulty recognizing and retaining main points Difficulty interpreting information Difficulty integrating information and drawing conclusions Difficulty detecting and comprehending inference	Explain stimuli by theme or gist; demonstrate appreciation of a character's motives, an implied outcome, or the moral of the story; identify essential, optional and irrelevant information; identify and explain absurdities that arise from contextual incongruence; recognize alternative interpretations of information

(contd)

Table 10.4 (contd)

Impairment	Suggested therapy activity
Word retrieval	
Reduced word association skills	Word association tasks; interpreting definitions; providing category names; comparing semantic items according to attributes; providing synonyms and antonyms
Organization of verbal expression	
Difficulty with efficient production of organized, meaningful verbal expression	Sequencing tasks; summarizing tasks; providing instructions to naïve listener; syntactic judgement tasks; story retelling; story generation; analysis and self-correction of recorded verbal expression
Organization of written expression	
Difficulty with efficient production of written expression	Sequencing tasks; summarizing tasks; providing step-by-step written instructions; short narrative production according to a narrative schema; self-correction of written information

To attain the intermediate goals that target certain functional skills, compensatory strategies and functional skills training can be used. Compensatory strategy training aims to teach the individual methods by which to overcome his/her deficits through the use of internal compensation. For example, the individual may be taught to use circumlocutions when frustrated by word-retrieval deficits, or ask for repetition or written information when they cannot understand detailed instructions. Functional skills training aims to improve the ability to perform a specific function through learning and repetition. Treatment is conducted within the functional communicative environment and is, by nature, activity based. For example, a functional skills task may involve specific training in the way to answer the telephone, convey feelings to a doctor, or operate a communication device.

While achievement of the immediate and intermediate goals will facilitate the realization of the long-term goal, environmental manipulation directly targets the long-term goal. This method endeavours to modify the physical and communicative environment so as to facilitate communicative success for the individual with MS. Such an intervention may include advising potential communicative partners as to the best methods of interaction, or altering the physical layout of a work office so that the person with MS is able to operate with limited distractions or extraneous noise.

Monitoring treatment outcome

Ongoing assessment of the communication ability of the person with MS is critical for a number of reasons. First, it is necessary for the clinician to monitor the success of the treatment strategies and make modifications accordingly. Secondly, the satisfaction of the stakeholders must be regularly surveyed to ensure the social value of the treatment and to promote continued motivation. Thirdly, the clinician must monitor for the effects of disease progression and appropriately alter the treatment programme in consultation with the stakeholders. Finally, it may be necessary to provide evidence of outcome success in order to provide clinical accountability and justify the ongoing financial support for the treatment programme.

The effectiveness of treatment can be determined by the achievement of the defined therapy goals. Documentation of outcome measurement can be incorporated into the therapy plan as illustrated in Figure 10.1. Outcome measures can include pre- and post-treatment test scores, surveys before, during and after treatment, or use of dedicated outcome scales. Enderby (1997) produced a series of outcome scales designed for use by speech-language pathologists to measure therapy outcome for a range of communication disorders. The scales are devised to assess outcome at the levels of impairment, disability, handicap and well-being. While there is a scale for dysphasia, there is no specific scale for acquired cognitive-communication disorders. The core scale, however, can be applied to any disorder and application of this scale to the cognitive-communication and functional communication disorders experienced by MS individuals is illustrated in the case studies presented below.

Promoting maintenance of communicative function

In degenerative diseases such as MS, the maintenance of functional skill may be a goal in itself. Even in cases where there is little apparent functional disability, a major concern for the individual may be to preserve their communicative skill for as long as possible. The speech-language pathologist may, therefore, be involved in promoting the maintenance of healthy communication skills. This may involve using challenging component process exercises and/or discussing and practising the use of compensatory strategies and environmental manipulations.

Group therapy is useful in the promotion of healthy communication function. Group situations provide opportunities for the MS individual to obtain feedback from significant communicative partners. Such feedback is important for the development of self-awareness and acceptance of functional abilities (Hartley, 1995). In addition, ongoing formal and informal group therapy provides opportunity for the practice of functional communication skills and permits the building of social relationships. Promoting a positive, understanding environment for communicative activity helps the individual with MS retain a positive attitude to meeting his/her communicative needs. An example of a maintenance programme is presented below in the case discussion of subject number 40.

Case examples

The following case examples provide illustrations of suggested treatment programmes for cognitive-communication disorders in MS patients. The cases have been drawn from a subject sample already documented in the literature (Lethlean and Murdoch, 1993, 1994a, 1997) and were chosen to represent the diversity of linguistic dysfunction reported in MS. Full personal details involving the nature of the communicative environments are not available for each case and, therefore, the everyday communicative demands placed on the individuals have been assumed for the purposes of illustration of intervention design.

Case 1 was introduced as Subject 23 in Chapter 7 and presents with a severe pervasive language impairment. Case 2 is Subject 24 who was described in Chapter 9 and represents the group of MS patients with substantial language deficits. Case 3 is Subject 20 from Chapter 9 and depicts a person with MS who has selective impairment of more complex cognitive-linguistic function. Case 4 was described as Subject 40 in Chapter 9 and portrays a person with MS who has maintained essentially normal linguistic and communicative status.

Case 1

Subject 23 is a 51-year-old woman with 16 years of education and a disease duration of 11 years. She resides in a nursing home and is confined to a wheelchair. At the time of testing she presented with visual disturbances, which interfered with the reading components of language testing. The linguistic deficits of Subject 23 were delineated using the test battery outlined in Chapter 9. Her performance on primary and higher-order tests of language function was well below that of normal control subjects and other MS subjects. Results indicated significant impairments of simple and complex auditory comprehension, visual naming, word retrieval, lexical-semantic manipulations and verbal formulation. It was the impression of the assessing clinician that the severely impaired performance by Subject 23 on the language tests may have been associated with the combined influence of considerable physical disability, visual impairment and institutionalization. In addition, it was considered that her difficulty with some of the tests possibly reflected the early stage of dementia; however, a full assessment of cognitive function was not available.

Subject 23, therefore, presents with marked linguistic and probable cognitive impairment which underpins considerable communication disability. After having identified this impairment, it is necessary to establish the communicative demands of Subject 23's environment. Given that she is physically dependent and resides in an institution, it can be assumed that the primary communicative partners are the staff caregivers, visitors and fellow residents. In designing a meaningful therapy programme it is necessary to establish, through consultation with Subject 23, the nature and importance of the communicative exchanges she engages in with each of these significant people. It is then important to determine whether and to what extent Subject 23's linguistic deficit impedes her functional communicative skill. The findings of the language assessment should then be interpreted in terms of the impact the linguistic deficiencies have on daily communicative function. The explanation serves as a basis for the rationale of the therapy programme and promotes acceptance of the intervention and motivation for participation. This explanation should be delivered not only to Subject 23 but also to her significant communicative partners.

Once the communicative needs have been identified and the extent of the communicative handicap observed, realistic treatment goals can be determined. Treatment goals need to be holistic, realistic and clearly stated and the time to reach them should be estimated. The goals of treatment need to be formulated by the clinician in consultation with Subject 23 and her consistent, significant communicative partners. In this case, where Subject 23 is experiencing widespread linguistic deficits associated with cognitive decline, it is likely that the emphasis on treatment should be on modification of the communicative environment and functional skills training. An example of a treatment programme for Subject 23 is illustrated in Figure 10.2. Treatment targeting specific linguistic operations, such as word-finding skills or auditory comprehension, may only be warranted if a cognitive assessment revealed adequate memory and attentional facility to learn and apply compensatory strategies.

The aim of modifying the communication environment for Subject 23 is to promote a desirable and comfortable situation in which she can achieve successful communication. Such an environment increases the likelihood of maintenance of communication and generalization of skill to other settings (Bourgeois, 1991). At the outset this may entail removing any frustrating physical barriers to communication. This involves examination of the orientation of furniture in the room so that spontaneous

Communication Therapy Programme

Name: Subject 23	Date:
Communication Environment: Home: Nursing Home Work: N/A	**Communication Partners:** Home: Staff; visitors - family and friends; other residents Work: N/A

Motor Speech: Mild dysarthria Vision: Impaired for reading	Long-term goal: To maintain current level of active participation in an assisted living situation. Maintain ability to communicate needs and interact socially with significant communicative partners.	Baseline Measure: 2*
Motor Control: Impaired fine motor Mobility: Wheelchair dependent	Suggested Intervention: Alter access to speaker phone; Alter orientation of wheelchair in living room to facilitate interaction; Counselling of staff and relatives.	Outcome Measure:

Immediate Goals	Baseline Measure	Suggested Intervention	Outcome Measure
1a. To be able to name or indicate body parts	4 ▲	Body part naming and indication; responsive naming; divergent naming tasks	
2a. To be able to identify multiple meanings of words	3 ▲	Identifying correct definitions; formulating definitions	
2b. To be able to identify main points of stories	3 ▲	Story retelling; summarizing; giving moral; giving titles and punchlines	

Intermediate Goals	Baseline Measure	Suggested Intervention	Outcome Measure
1. To be able to describe symptoms to doctors or care-giver	2 ◆	Role-play; rehearsal	
2. To be able to maintain attention to and comprehension of conversations with visitors	2 ◆	Teaching strategies to seek clarification or repetition of information; Counselling of relatives and friends re: strategies to facilitate comprehension in conversation	

Treatment Schedule: 2 hours/week

Maintenance Schedule: group therapy 1 hour/week

* Score relates to the Handicap Level of the 'Core Scale' of Therapy Outcome Measures (Enderby, 1997) : 2 = Some integration, value and autonomy in one setting

♦ Score relates to the Disability Level of the 'Core Scale' of Therapy Outcome Measures (Enderby, 1997) : 2 = Can undertake some part of task but needs a high level of support to complete

▲ Score relates to the Impairment Level of the 'Core Scale' of Therapy Outcome Measures (Enderby, 1997) : 3 = Moderate presentation; 4 = Just below normal/mild presentation

Figure 10.2 Section of a communication therapy plan for Subject 23 (Case 1)

communicative situations are not thwarted by an inability to see, hear, or move close to a communicative partner. In addition, the communicative expectations of the environment may need to be modified. Subject 23's carers and other significant communicative partners need to be aware of the limitations on communication experienced by Subject 23 and alter their expectations accordingly. They may need to be instructed as to how to best simplify their verbal messages so that accurate auditory processing is possible. In addition, they may be taught strategies to provide Subject 23 with external cues to facilitate word retrieval or the formulation of an effective circumlocution. In essence, the communicative environment needs to foster communication and provide naturally occurring reinforcers so that maintenance of communication is achieved.

With intervention strategies in place, it is necessary to monitor their effectiveness and modify accordingly. Valid outcome measures will ensure the ongoing satisfaction of the MS patient and other stakeholders in the therapy programme.

Case 2

Case 2 is Subject 24, a 59-year-old female with 10 years of schooling, who was first diagnosed with MS at 26 years of age. She is now wheelchair dependent and living in her own home, but requires nursing assistance for daily living tasks. Subject 24 was assessed on the language battery outlined in Chapter 9. Results of her performance on tests of basic language function indicated intact simple visual naming, verbal expression, repetition, and reading skills. She presented, however, with deficits in right and left tactile naming, writing, and repetition of digits in reverse order. Examination of more complex language functions revealed that Subject 24 had considerable difficulty with verbal language comprehension and expression. She was found to have difficulty with word retrieval, formulation and monitoring of complex expression, semantic organization, and comprehension of complex linguistic structures.

The first step in designing a treatment programme for Subject 24 is to identify the communication demands of her environment. This entails establishing the 'who, what, when and where' of the communicative interactions that are important to Subject 24. Given that Subject 24 resides at home it may be assumed that she has a variety of communicative opportunities available to her and is likely to have contact not only with family and/or care-givers, but also with members of the general public. It is then necessary to determine the impact that the linguistic limitations identified on testing have on Subject 24's ability to meet those communicative needs. This is done by closely examining the test behaviour in conjunction with observational assessment and consultation with Subject 24 and her significant communicative partners.

Examination of the test results indicate that Subject 24 has adequate linguistic skills to engage in simple communicative interactions, but experiences sufficient reduction in linguistic proficiency to affect the achievement of high-level verbal communication. For example, it could be assumed that Subject 24's difficulty with efficient word retrieval and verbal formulation would limit her ability to describe acontextual situations, to explain abstract notions involving human feelings and reactions, and to express herself adequately in a pressured or non-familiar environment. There is also evidence on assessment that Subject 24 has difficulty comprehending inferred information, metaphoric expression and complex syntactic structures. From this information it may be predicted that Subject 24 could have difficulty integrating information in a story or movie, following lengthy or complex directions, or detecting subtle messages or connotative meanings in conversations with others. An intervention programme should establish if such functional consequences do occur and to what extent they impact on quality of life for Subject 24. After consultation with Subject 24 and her significant communicative partners, therapy targets should be designed.

The initial step in achieving the therapy targets is to ensure that Subject 24 is aware of the nature of the linguistic deficits which underpin the difficulties she may be experiencing with communication. With a metacognitive understanding of her deficits Subject 24 would be able to participate in determining therapy goals and may be more likely to be motivated to achieve them. In this case, four types of intervention (Hartley, 1995) could be applied simultaneously, namely, component process retraining, environmental manipulation, compensatory strategy training, and functional skills training. An example of a section of a communication therapy programme for Subject 24 is illustrated in Figure 10.3. Component process retraining could be applied to deficits in auditory processing. Subject 24 could be required to attend to and accurately process an increasingly complex series of commands or statements. She should be instructed to detect and attend to the salient information. Simultaneously, compensatory strategies such as requesting repetitions or slower delivery, self-repetition of the instruction, and visual imagery, could be taught and applied.

Compensatory strategy training could also be used to facilitate word retrieval. Encouraging the use of circumlocution to effectively communicate the salient semantic elements of the unretrieved lexical item would be advantageous. Similarly, the use of semantic associations could effectively prime the retrieval of the desired lexical item.

Certain communicative situations, which have been identified as important and difficult for Subject 24, could be analysed for the purposes of functional skills training. This process entails delineating

Communication Therapy Programme

Name: Subject 24	Date:

Communication Partners:
Home: Husband, daughter, son-in-law, friends, neighbour, visiting nurses, neighbourhood retailers
Work: N/A

Communication Environment:
Home: Living at home with ADL assistance
Work: N/A

Motor Speech: Mild dysarthria

Vision: Some difficulty reading

Long-term goal: To maintain living in home environment and current satisfactory level of verbal communication	Baseline Measure: 3*
Suggested Intervention: Counselling re: communication limitations; Counselling of significant others and instruction re: assisting comprehension.	Outcome Measure:

Motor Control: Impaired fine-motor – difficulty writing

Mobility: wheelchair dependent

Immediate Goals	Baseline Measure	Suggested Intervention	Outcome Measure
1a. Able to comprehend short paragraphs	3 ▲	Preview material and identify central ideas or themes or central ideas; answer questions; summarize information, detect main points. Increase length of stimulus; Practise looking at person, preparing to listen; use active thinking – mentally repeating main points; acknowledge comprehension;	
1b. Improve listening behaviour	3 ▲		
1c. Able to organize and produce relevant points ...	3 ▲		

Intermediate Goals	Baseline Measure	Suggested Intervention	Outcome Measure
1. To be able to participate in conversation with a group of 2 or more	3 ◆	Practice of targeted skills in simulated situations; Counselling of communicative partners re: checking for comprehension, paraphasing, providing clarification ...	

Intermediate Goals	Baseline Measure	Suggested Intervention	Outcome Measure	Immediate Goals	Baseline Measure	Suggested Intervention	Outcome Measure
						reinforce speaker; seek clarification.	
						Formulate messages in complex sentences containing cause-effect, conditional, spatial, or temporal relationships....	

Treatment Schedule: 3 hours/week

Maintenance Schedule: Group therapy 1 hour/week

* Score relates to the Handicap Level of the 'Core Scale' of Therapy Outcome Measures (Enderby, 1997) : 3 = Integrated, valued and autonomous in limited number of settings

◆ Score relates to the Disability Level of the 'Core Scale' of Therapy Outcome Measures (Enderby, 1997) : 3 = Can undertake task/function in familiar situation but requires some verbal/physical assistance

▲ Score relates to the Impairment Level of the 'Core Scale' of Therapy Outcome Measures (Enderby, 1997) : 3 = Moderate presentation

Figure 10.3 Section of a communication therapy programme for Subject 24 (Case 2)

the 'script' of the situation by noting the type of communicative acts and content. Once the nature of the troublesome communication exchange has been broken down it can be rehearsed acontextually. The ultimate goal is to achieve generalization of the skills rehearsed so that more successful communication can be achieved in the real life situation.

Environmental manipulation is also required to enhance Subject 24's communicative opportunities and success. This may involve modification of the physical environment in order to facilitate interpersonal interaction. It could also involve informing Subject 24's significant communicative partners of the nature of her linguistic impairment and ensuring that they are aware of her limitations. The therapist can then give the communicative partners strategies to help facilitate effective communication with Subject 24. For example, they may be encouraged to simplify verbal instruction, repeat important information, or reduce the rate of delivery when telling a story or giving a long explanation. In addition, it may be recommended that they seek clarification from Subject 24 that she has understood the information that has been delivered. Communicative partners can also assist Subject 24 when she experiences frustration with lexical retrieval by providing her with some external prompts.

All treatment goals require ongoing monitoring and alteration. Success should be measured by the qualitative improvements in the efficiency with which Subject 24 can meet the communicative requirements of her daily life.

Case 3

Case 3 is Subject 20 who is a 57-year-old male with 10 years of education, who was reported in Chapter 9 as having selective impairment of cognitive-linguistic function. He is independently mobile and living at home. Neuropsychological evaluation revealed that at the time of testing Subject 20 had experienced deterioration in the cognitive processes of attention, concentration, memory and organizational abilities. Language testing revealed that Subject 20 had a normal capacity with primary linguistic operations, but had selective impairments of more complex linguistic processes. Difficulties were experienced with word retrieval and identification and explanation of the critical semantic elements of words. Verbal formulation of complex descriptions and explanations was also impaired. Only minor difficulty was experienced with auditory processing.

As with cases 1 and 2, the impact of these identified deficiencies on Subject 20's communicative environment needs to be established. In accordance with the philosophy of 'life-style' therapy, this has to be done in consultations with Subject 20 and any other stakeholders. Likewise, the determination of therapy goals must be conducted in consultation with all of the significant communicators. A sample of possible therapy goals and treatment plan for Subject 20 is illustrated in Figure 10.4.

Subject 20 must first acquire metacognitive awareness of the nature of his linguistic impairments and the consequential handicap in communication that they cause. Given that the linguistic deficits are selective and involve higher-order skills, some degree of component process training may be warranted. Treatment may entail exercises requiring lexical retrieval and semantic judgement. Compensatory strategies and environmental manipulations that maximize communicative opportunities and promote successful communication would be designed.

Given his history of slow cognitive decline, Subject 20 would require careful ongoing monitoring and counselling regarding the possible deterioration in linguistic ability and communicative effectiveness. With continued monitoring, alterations in the therapy goals and intervention techniques could be justified.

Case 4

Case 4 is Subject 40, who is a 25-year-old female with 10 years of education. She is independently mobile and living at home. Despite having experienced a global decrease in higher cognitive functions since the onset of MS, Subject 40 presented with essentially near normal status on tests of language function. Her performance, however, was marked by some qualitative distinctions. While Subject 40 had good naming and word retrieval ability, adequate verbal reasoning techniques, and intact auditory comprehension, she experienced some mild expressive language deficits.

While most clinicians would not retain Subject 40 on their caseload, attention to her communicative needs is indeed warranted and intervention should not be overlooked. An example of an intervention plan is illustrated in Figure 10.5. With her youth and ability to operate well in the community, it is likely that she is experiencing a multitude of daily interactional situations. A speech-language assessment of Subject 40 should extend to documentation of the type of communicative activities she engages in and the importance she places on them.

Subject 40 would benefit from periodic therapy sessions that monitor linguistic ability and communication skills and offer counselling. Group therapy may also provide Subject 40 with opportunities to maintain self-awareness and confidence in her interactional abilities through feedback from friends. Counselling should involve informing Subject 40 of the possibility that she may encounter difficulty in communication at some future point and should describe the likely nature of such difficulties. By establishing such a relationship between the therapist and patient,

Communication Therapy Programme

Name: Subject 20	Date:

Communication Environment:
Home: Living at home independently

Work: N/A

Communication Partners:
Home: visitors - children, grandchildren, friends, community members
Work: N/A

	Baseline Measure	Outcome Measure
Motor Speech: WNL Vision: Impaired for reading		
Long-term goal: Maintain independent functional status at home and in the community	Baseline Measure: 4*	Outcome Measure:
Motor Control: Impaired fine motor Mobility: Independently mobile		
Suggested Intervention: Counselling - Subject 20 and significant others; Maintenance therapy - see immediate goals		Outcome Measure

Intermediate Goals	Baseline Measure	Suggested Intervention	Outcome Measure	Immediate Goals	Baseline Measure	Suggested Intervention	Outcome Measure
1. Able to organize shopping list for phone order	4◆	Functional skills training; Compensatory strategy training		1a. Improve word retrieval	3–4▲	Semantic categorization tasks; divergent word finding tasks.	
2. Able to formulate verbal expression for conversational purposes	4◆	Counselling re: attention focusing strategies.....		2a. Improve semantic and pragmatic consistency of sentence production	3–4▲	Semantic judgement tasks; formulation tasks given main words and contexts; monitoring consistency	
				2b. Reduce irrelevancy and tangential information....	3▲	Identify main points of information; summarizing tasks; revision and self-monitoring exercises....	

Treatment Schedule: 2 hours/week

Maintenance Schedule: group therapy 1 × week

* Score relates to the Handicap Level of the 'Core Scale' of Therapy Outcome Measures (Enderby, 1997) : 4 = Occasionally some restriction in autonomy, integration, or role

♦ Score relates to the Disability Level of the 'Core Scale' of Therapy Outcome Measures (Enderby, 1997) : 4= Requires some minor assistance occasionally or extra time to complete task

▲ Score relates to the Impairment Level of the 'Core Scale' of Therapy Outcome Measures (Enderby, 1997) : 3 = Moderate presentation; 4 = Just below normal/mild presentation

Figure 10.4 Section of a communication therapy plan for Subject 20 (Case 3)

Communication Therapy Programme	
Name: Subject 40	Date:
Communication Environment: Home: Independent Work: Receptionist	Communication Partners: Home: Spouse, visitors - family members and friends Work: Office workers - senior and junior staff; customers

		Baseline Measure:
Motor Speech: WNL Vision: WNL	Long-term goal: To maintain independence at home and at the work place; To maintain friendships with peers	Baseline Measure: 5*
Motor Control: WNL Mobility: Independently mobile	Suggested Intervention: Counselling of Subject 40 and significant others re: disease progression and effects on communicative skill. Maintenance program	Outcome Measure:

Intermediate Goals	Baseline Measure	Suggested Intervention	Outcome Measure	Immediate Goals	Baseline Measure	Suggested Intervention	Outcome Measure
1. Gain understanding of possible deterioration in linguistic skill.		Interactive counselling sessions; written information.		1a. Will recognize aspects of communicative function which are vulnerable		Information-giving sessions and reviews; Ongoing assessment of function	
				1b. Will learn strategies to monitor communicative effectiveness.		Counselling and skills training in simulated situation.	

Treatment Schedule: Maintenance

Maintenance Schedule: Review and counselling 1 × 3 months

* Score relates to the Handicap Level of the 'Core Scale' of Therapy Outcome Measures (Enderby, 1997) : 5 = Integrated, valued, occupies appropriate role

Figure 10.5 Section of a communication therapy plan for Subject 40 (Case 4)

natural and effective compensatory strategies for any communication disabilities which do occur can be implemented early. In this way, the observable functional deficit is minimized and Subject 40 would be better able to maintain her communicative status, social adjustment and quality of life.

Conclusion

The existence of language deficits in MS is becoming widely acknowledged. Clinicians involved in the rehabilitation of MS patients may recognize a functional communication impairment and the need to assess their patients on tests involving higher-order language function. Therapeutic intervention with degenerative diseases, such as MS, should largely focus on teaching compensatory strategies and modification of the environment so as to promote maximum function and minimize disability and communication handicap. The process of this intervention involves identifying the communicative needs and the impact of the linguistic deficits on the ability of the person to meet those needs. This is followed by establishing therapy goals and implementing intervention, the success of which must be closely monitored.

For this therapy to achieve success, it is essential that the person whose functional status is compromised is integral to treatment design, implementation and monitoring. The ultimate goal of therapy should be to facilitate the individual's ability to participate in his/her everyday activities and maintain psychosocial well-being through the prevention of social isolation.

Appendix
Component process treatment material sources

Hahn SE, Klein ER (1989) Focus on Function: Retraining for the Communicatively Impaired Client. Arizona: Communication Skill Builders.

Holloran SM, Bressler EJ (1983) Cognitive Reorganisation: A Stimulus Handbook. Texas: Pro-ed.

Lazzari AM, Peters PM (1989) HELP 4 Handbook of Exercises for Language Processing. East Moline: LinguiSystems.

Tomlin KJ (1993) WALC 1 Workbook of Activities for Language and Cognition: For Lower Levels of Cognition and Aphasia. East Moline: LinguiSystems.

Tomlin KJ (1993) WALC 3 Workbook of Activities for Language and Cognition: Word Finding, Organization, Reasoning, Visual Tasks. East Moline: LinguiSystems.

References

Abbs JH, De Paul R (1989) Assessment of dysarthria: the critical prerequisite to treatment. In Leahy MM (ed.) Disorders of Communication: The Science of Intervention. London: Taylor and Francis: 206–27.

Abbs JH, Hartman DE, Vishwanat B (1987) Orofacial motor control impairment in Parkinson's disease. Neurology 37: 394–8.

Acheson E (1985) The epidemiology of multiple sclerosis. In Matthews WB (ed.) McAlpine's Multiple Sclerosis. London: Churchill Livingstone: 3–27.

Achiron A, Ziu I, Djaldetti R, Goldberg H, Kuritzky A, Melamed E (1992) Aphasia in multiple sclerosis: clinical and radiographic correlations. Neurology 42: 2195–7.

Ackerman H, Hertrich I (1993) Speech rate and rhythm in cerebellar dysarthria: an acoustic analysis of syllabic timing. Folia Phoniatrica et Logopaedica 46: 70–8.

Ackerman H, Ziegler W (1991) Cerebellar voice tremor: an acoustic analysis. Journal of Neurology, Neurosurgery, and Psychiatry 54: 74–6.

Ackerman H, Ziegler W (1994) Acoustic analysis of vocal instability in cerebellar dysfunctions. Annals of Otology, Rhinology and Laryngology 103: 98–104.

Adams SG (1994) Accelerating speech in a case of hypokinetic dysarthria: descriptions and treatment. In Till JA, Yorkston KM, Beukelman DR (eds.) Motor Speech Disorders: Advances in Assessment and Treatment. Baltimore: Paul H Brookes Publishing Co: 213–28.

Adams SG, Lang AE (1992) Can the Lombard effect be used to improve low voice intensity in Parkinson's disease? European Journal of Disorders of Communication 27: 121–7.

Alexander MP, LoVerme SR (1980) Aphasia after left hemisphere intracerebral haemorrhage. Neurology 30: 1193–1202.

Alexander GE, DeLong MR, Strick PL (1986) Parallel organisation of functionally segregated circuits linking basal ganglia and cortex. Annual Review of Neuroscience 9: 357–81.

Alexander MP, Naeser MA, Palumbo CL (1987) Correlations of subcortical CT lesion sites and aphasia profiles. Brain 110: 961–91.

Allen CM (1970) Treatment of nonfluent speech resulting from neurological disease – treatment of dysarthria. British Journal of Disorders of Communication 5: 3–5.

Allen IV (1991) Pathology of multiple sclerosis. In Matthews WB, Compston A, Allen IV, Martyn CN (eds.) McAlpine's Multiple Sclerosis, 2nd edn. New York: Churchill Livingstone: 341–78.

American Speech-Language-Hearing Association (ASHA) (1987) Report of the sub-committee on language and cognition: the role of the speech-language pathologist in the habilitation and rehabilitation of cognitively impaired individuals. American Speech and Hearing Association Journal 29: 53–5.

American Speech-Language-Hearing Association (ASHA) (1990) Guidelines for speech-language pathologists serving persons with language, socio-communicative, and or cognitive-communicative impairments. American Speech and Hearing Association Journal 32: 85–92.

Anzola GP, Bevilaqual L, Cappa SF, Capra R, Faglia L, Farina E, Frisoni G, Mariani C, Pasolini MP, Vignolo LA (1990) Neuropsychological assessment in patients with relapsing remitting multiple sclerosis and mild functional impairment: correlation with MRI. Journal of Neurology, Neurosurgery & Psychiatry 153: 142–5.

Arnott WL, Jordan FM, Murdoch BE, Lethlean JB (1997) Narrative discourse in multiple sclerosis: an investigation of conceptual structure. Aphasiology 11: 969–91.

Aronson AE (1985) Clinical Voice Disorders, 2nd edn. New York: Thieme Inc.

Aten JL (1994) Functional communication treatment. In Chapey R (ed.) Language Intervention Strategies in Adult Aphasia, 3rd edn. Baltimore: Williams & Wilkins: 292–303.

Baken RJ (1987) Clinical Measurement of Speech and Voice. Boston MA: College-Hill Press.

Baken RJ, Cavallo SA, Weissman KL (1979) Chest wall movements prior to phonation. Journal of Speech and Hearing Research 22: 862–72.

Baldwin R, Luce T, Readence O (1982) The impact of subschema on metaphorical processing. Reading Research Quarterly 4: 528–43.

Barkhof F, Tas MW, Frequin ST, Sheltens P, Hommes OR, Nauta JJP, Valk J (1994) Limited duration of the effect of methylprednisolone on changes on MRI in multiple sclerosis. Neuroradiology 36: 382–7.

Barlow SM, Abbs JH (1983) Force transducers for the evaluation of labial, lingual and mandibular motor impairments. Journal of Speech and Hearing Research 26: 616–21.

Barlow SM, Burton M (1988) Orofacial force control impairments in brain-injured adults. Association for Research in Otolaryngology Abstracts 11: 218.

Barlow SM, Netsell R (1986) Differential fine force control of the upper and lower lips. Journal of Speech and Hearing Research 29: 163–9.

Barnes D, Munro PM, Youl BD, Prineas JW, McDonald WI (1991) The longlasting multiple sclerosis lesion: a quantitative MRI and electron microscopic study. Brain 114: 1271–80.

Bastian RW (1987) Laryngeal image biofeedback for voice disorder patients. Journal of Voice 1: 279–82.

Batchelor JR (1985) Immunological and pathological aspects. In Matthews WB (ed.) McAlpine's Multiple Sclerosis. London: Churchill Livingstone: 281–300.

Bauer HJ, Hanefeld FA (1993) Multiple Sclerosis: Its Impact from Childhood to Old Age. London: W B Saunders Company Ltd.

Baumhefner RW, Tourtellotte WW, Syndulko K, Waluch V, Ellison GW, Meyers LW, Cohen SN, Osborne M, Shapshak P (1990) Quantitative multiple sclerosis plaque assessment with magnetic resonance imaging: its correlation with clinical parameters, evoked potentials, and intra-blood brain barrier IgG synthesis. Archives of Neurology 47: 19–26.

Bayles KA, Boone DR (1982) The potential of language tasks for identifying senile dementia. Journal of Speech and Hearing Disorders 47: 210–17.

Bayles KA, Tomoeda CK (1983) Confrontation naming impairment in dementia. Brain and Language 19: 114

Bayles KA, Tomoeda CK (1991) Arizona Battery for Communication Disorders of Dementia Test Manual. Tucson AZ: Canyonlands.Beach CM (1991) The interpretation of prosodic patterns at points of syntactic structure ambiguity: evidence for cue trading relations. Journal of Memory and Language 30: 644–63.

Beatty WW, Monson N (1989) Lexical processing in Parkinson's disease and multiple sclerosis. Journal of Geriatric Psychiatry and Neurology 2: 145–52.

Beatty WW, Monson N (1990) Semantic priming in multiple sclerosis. Bulletin of Psychonomic Society 28: 397–400.

Beatty W W, Goodkin D E, Monson N, Beatty PA, Hertsgaard D (1988) Anterograde and retrograde amnesia in patients with chronic progressive multiple sclerosis. Archives of Neurology 45: 611–19.

Beatty WW, Monson N, Goodkin DE (1989) Access to semantic memory in Parkinson's disease and multiple sclerosis. Journal of Geriatric Psychiatry & Neurology 2: 153–62.

Beatty WW, Goodkin DE, Monson N, Beatty PA (1989). Cognitive disturbances in patients with relapsing-remitting multiple sclerosis. Archives of Neurology 46: 1113–19.

Beatty WW, Goodkin DE, Hertsgaard D, Monson N (1990) Clinical and demographic predictors of cognitive performance in multiple sclerosis: do diagnostic type, disease, duration and disability matter? Archives of Neurology 47: 305–8.

Bellaire K, Yorkston KM, Beukelman DR (1986) Modification of breath patterning to increase naturalness of a mildly dysarthric speaker. Journal of Communication Disorders 19: 271–80.

Bennett TL (1989) Neuropsychological impairment in a case of juvenile multiple sclerosis. International Journal of Clinical Neuropsychology 11: 182–6.

Bennett T, Dittmar C, Raubach S (1991) Multiple sclerosis: cognitive deficits and rehabilitation strategies. Cognitive Rehabilitation 9: 18–23.

Benton AL, Hamsher K (1983) Multilingual Aphasia Examination, rev edn. Iowa City: AJA Associates.

Bernstein DK (1987) Figurative language: assessment strategies and implications for intervention. Folia Phoniatrica 39: 130–44.

Berry WR (1983) Treatment of hypokinetic dysarthria. In Perkins WR (ed.) Current Therapy of Communication Disorders: Dysarthria and Apraxia. New York: Thieme-Stratton: 91–9.

Berry WR, Goshorn EL (1983) Immediate visual feedback in the treatment of ataxic dysarthria: a case study. In Berry WR (ed.) Clinical dysarthria. San Diego: College-Hill Press: 253–65.

Berry WR, Sanders WB (1983) Environmental education: the universal management approach for adults with dysarthria. In Berry WR (ed.) Clinical Dysarthria. Boston: College-Hill Press: 203–16.

Beukelman DR, Mirenda P (1992) Augmentative and Alternative Communication: Management of Severe Communication Disorders in Children and Adults. Baltimore: Paul H Brookes.

Beukelman DR, Yorkston KM (1978) Communication options for patients with brain stem lesions. Archives of Physical Medicine and Rehabilitation 59: 337–40.

Beukelman DR, Kraft GH, Freal J (1985) Expressive communication disorders in persons with multiple sclerosis: a survey. Archives of Physical Medicine and Rehabilitation 66: 675–7.

Beukelman DR, Yorkston KM, Tice B (1988) Pacer/Tally. Tucson: Communication Skill Builders.

Blackwood HD, La Pointe LL, Holtzapple P, Pohlman K, Graham LF (1991) Lexical-semantic abilities of individuals with multiple sclerosis and aphasia. In Prescott RE (ed.) Clinical Aphasiology. Austin TX: Pro-Ed: 121–7.

Blanken G, Dittmann J, Haas CJ, Wallesch CW (1987) Spontaneous speech in senile dementia and aphasia: implications for a neurolinguistic model of language production. Cognition 23: 247–74.

Bless DM (1988) Voice disorders in the adult: treatment. In Yoder DE, Kent RD (eds) Decision Making in Speech-language Pathology. Philadelphia: BC Decker: 140–3.

Blonder LX, Gur RE, Gur RC, Saykin AJ, Hurtig HI (1989) Neuropsychological functioning in hemiparkinsonism. Brain and Cognition 9: 244–57.

Bock TK (1982) Toward a cognitive psychology of syntax: information processing contributions to sentence formulation. Psychological Review 89: 1–47.

Boone DR (1977) The Voice and Voice Therapy, 2nd edn. Englewood Cliffs: Prentice-Hall.

Boone DR, McFarlane SC (1988) The Voice and Voice Therapy, 4th edn. Englewood Cliffs: Prentice-Hall.

Boren HG, Kory RC, Synder JC (1966) The Veterans Administration-Army co-operative study of pulmonary function II: the lung volume and its subdivisions in normal men. American Journal of Medicine 41: 96–114.

Bougle F, Ryalls J, Le Dorze G (1995) Improving fundamental frequency modulation in head trauma patients: a preliminary comparison of speech-language therapy conducted with and without IBM's Speech Viewer. Folia Phoniatrica Logopedia 47: 24–32.

Bourgeois MS (1991) Communication treatment for adults with dementia. Journal of Speech and Hearing Research 34: 831–44.

Brancewicz TM, Reich AR (1989) Speech rate reduction and nasality in normal speakers. Journal of Speech and Hearing Research 32: 837–48.

Brooks DJ, Leenders KL, Head G, Marshall J, Legg NJ, Jones T (1984) Studies on regional cerebral oxygen utilisation and cognitive function in MS. Journal of Neurology, Neurosurgery & Psychiatry 47: 1182–91.

Brookshire RH, Nicholas LE (1993) Discourse Comprehension Test. Tuscon AZ: Communication Skill Builders.

Brown JR, Darley FL, Aronson AE (1970) Ataxic dysarthria. International Journal of Neurology 7: 302–18.

Bryan K (1989) The Right Hemisphere Language Battery. Southampton: Far Communications.

Buder EH, Kent RD, Kent JF, Milenkovic P, Workinger M (1996) FORMOFFA: An automated formant, moment, fundamental frequency, amplitude analysis of normal and disordered speech. Clinical Linguistics and Phonetics 10(1): 31–54.

Burgess C, Simpson G B (1988) Cerebral hemispheric mechanisms in the retrieval of ambiguous word meanings. Brain Language 33: 86–103.

Butters N, Granholm E, Salmon DP, Grant I, Wolfe J (1987) Episodic and semantic memory: A comparison of amnesic and demented patients. Journal of Clinical and Experimental Neuropsychology 9: 479–97.

Buyse B, Demedts M, Meekers J, Vandegaer L, Rochette F, Kerkhofs L (1997) Respiratory dysfunction in multiple sclerosis: a prospective analysis of 60 patients. European Respiratory Journal 10: 139–45.

Byrd M (1988) Adult age differences in the ability to comprehend ambiguous sentences. Language and Communication 8: 135–46.

Caine ED, Bamford KA, Schiffer RB, Shoulson I, Levy S, (1986) A controlled neuropsychological comparison of Huntington's disease and multiple sclerosis. Archives of Neurology 43: 249–54.

Caligiuri MP, Murry T (1983) The use of visual feedback to enhance prosodic control in dysarthria. In Berry WR (ed.) Clinical Dysarthria 267–82 San Diego: College-Hill Press: 267–82.

Callanan MM, Logsdail S, Ron MA, Warrington EK (1989) Cognitive impairment in patients with clinically isolated lesions of the type seen in multiple sclerosis: a psychometric and MRI study. Brain 112: 361–74.

Cappa SF, Vignolo LA (1979) 'Transcortical' features of aphasia following left thalamic haemorrhage. Cortex 15: 121–30.

Capra R, Marciano N, Vignolo LA, Chiesa A, Gasparotti R (1992) Gadolinium – penetetic acid magnetic resonance imaging in patients with relapsing remitting multiple sclerosis. Archives of Neurology 49: 687–9.

Carpenter RJ, McDonald TJ, Howard FM (1978) The otolaryngologic presentation of amyotrophic lateral sclerosis. Otolaryngology 86: 479–84.

Cavallo SA, Baken RJ (1985) Prephonatory laryngeal and chest wall dynamics. Journal of Speech and Hearing Research 28: 79–87.

Charcot J-M (1877) Lectures on the Diseases of the Nervous System. London: New Sydenham Society.

Charcot J-M (1877) Leçons sur les maladies du système nerveux I. Paris: Adrien Delahaye.

Chenery HJ, Murdoch BE (1994) The production of narrative discourse in response to animation in persons with dementia of the Alzheimer's type: preliminary findings. Aphasiology 8: 159–71.

Chertkow H, Bub D (1990) Semantic memory loss in dementia of the Alzheimer's type: what do various measures measure? Brain 113: 397–417.

Cobble ND, Bontke CF, Brandstater ME, Horn LJ (1991) Rehabilitation in brain disorders: three intervention strategies. Archives of Physical Medicine and Rehabilitation 72: S324–7.

Coelho CA, DeRuyter F, Stein M (1996) Treatment efficacy: cognitive-communicative disorders resulting from traumatic brain injury in adults. Journal of Speech and Hearing Research 39: 5–17.

Colton RH, Casper JK (1996) Understanding voice problems: a physiological perspective for diagnosis and treatment. Baltimore: Williams & Wilkins.

Colton RH, Conture EG (1990) Problems and pitfalls of electroglottography. Journal of Voice 4: 10–24.

Compston A (1994) The epidemiology of multiple sclerosis: principles, achievements and recommendations: Annals of Neurology 36 (Suppl. 2): 211–17.

Cook SD, Rohowsky-Kochan C, Bansil S, Dowling PC (1995) Evidence for multiple sclerosis as an infectious disease. Acta Neurologica Scandinavica 161: 34–42.

Crosson B (1985) Subcortical functions in language: a working model. Brain and Language 25: 257–92.

Crow E, Enderby P (1989) The effects of an alphabet chart on the speaking rate and intelligibility of speakers with dysarthria. In Yorkston KM, Beukelman DR (eds.) Recent Advances in Clinical Dysarthria. San Diego: College-Hill Press: 99–107.

Cummings JL, Benson DF (1988) Psychological dysfunction accompanying subcortical dementias. Annual Review of Medicine 39: 53–61.

Damasio AR, Damasio H, Rizzo M, Varney N, Gersh F (1982) Aphasia with nonhaemorrhagic lesions in the basal ganglia and internal capsule. Archives of Neurology 39: 15–20.

Darley FL, Aronson AE, Brown JR (1969a) Clusters of deviant speech dimensions in the dysarthria. Journal of Speech and Hearing Research 12: 462–96.

Darley FL, Aronson AE, Brown JR (1969b) Differential diagnostic patterns of dysarthria. Journal of Speech and Hearing Research 12: 246–69.

Darley FL, Brown JR, Goldstein NP (1972) Dysarthria in multiple sclerosis. Journal of Speech and Hearing Research 15: 229–45.

Day TJ, Fisher AG, Mastaglia FL (1987) Alexia with agraphia in multiple sclerosis. Journal of the Neurological Sciences 78: 343–8.

Dennis M, Barnes MA (1990) Knowing the meaning, getting the point, bridging the gap, and carrying the message: aspects of discourse following closed head injury in childhood and adolescence. Brain and Language 39: 428–46.

Dennis M, Lovett M W (1990) Discourse ability in children after brain damage. In Joanette Y, Brownell HH (eds.) Discourse Ability and Brain Damage. New York: Springer-Verlag: 199–221.

De Paul R, Brooks BR (1993) Multiple orofacial indices in amotrophic lateral sclerosis. Journal of Speech and Hearing Research 36: 1158–67.

De Paul R, Abbs JH, Caligiuri MP, Gracco VL, Brooks BR (1988) Hypoglossal, trigeminal, and facial motorneuron involvement in amyotrophic lateral sclerosis. Neurology 38: 281–3.

De Souza L (1990) Multiple Sclerosis: Approaches to Management. London: Chapman & Hall.

Dick G (1976) The etiology of multiple sclerosis. Central African Journal of Medicine 23: 129–30.

Diller, L (1987) Neuropsychological rehabilitation. In Meier MJ, Benton AL Diller L (eds.) Neuropsychological Rehabilitation. London: Churchill-Livingstone: 1–17.

Dongilli PA (1994) Semantic context and speech intelligibility. In Till JA, Yorkston KM, Beukelman DR (eds.) Motor Speech Disorders: Advances in Assessment and Treatment. Baltimore: Paul H Brookes Publishing Company: 175–92.

Draizar D (1984) Clinical EMG feedback in motor speech disorders. Archives of Physical Medicine and Rehabilitation 65: 481–4.

Duffy JR (1995) Motor Speech Disorders: Substrates, Differential Diagnosis, and Management. Baltimore: Mosby-Year Book.

Dworkin JP, Johns DF (1980) Management of velopharyngeal incompetence in dysarthria: An historical review. Clinical Otolaryngology 5: 61–74.

Ebers GC (1992) Infections and demyelinating disease: Editorial overview. Current Opinions in Neurology and Neurosurgery 5: 173–4.

Ebers GC (1994) Treatment of multiple sclerosis. The Lancet 343: 275–9.

Ebers GC, Bulman DE, Sadovnick AD, Paty DW, Warren S, Hader W, Murray TJ, Seland P, Duquette P, Grey T, Nelson R, Nicolle M, Brunet D (1986) A population-based study of multiple sclerosis in twins. New England Journal of Medicine 315: 1638–42.

Ehrlich JS (1988) Selective characteristics of narrative discourse in head-injured and normal adults. Journal of Communication Disorders 21: 1–9.

Ehrlich J, Barry P (1989) Rating communication behaviours in the head-injured adult. Brain Injury 3: 193–8.

Ehrlich J, Sipes A (1985) Group treatment of communication skills for head trauma patients. Cognitive Rehabilitation 3: 32–7.

Eisen A (1983) Neurophysiology in multiple sclerosis. Neurologic Clinics 1: 615

Enderby PM (1983) Frenchay Dysarthria Assessment. San Diego: College-Hill Press.

Enderby PM (1997) Therapy Outcome Measures (TOM) Speech and Language Therapy: User's Manual. London: Singular Publishing Group Inc.

Enderby P, Hathorn IS, Servant S (1984) The use of intra-oral appliances in the management of acquired velopharyngeal disorders. British Dental Journal 157: 157–9.

Erickson RP, Lie MR, Wineinger MA (1989) Rehabilitation in multiple sclerosis. Mayo Clinic Proceedings 64: 818–28.

Eriksson A (1991) Aspects of Swedish speech rhythm. Dissertation Department of Linguistics, Göteborg University, Göteborg, Sweden.

Espir MLE, Watkins SM, Smith HV (1966) Paroxysmal dysarthria and other transient neurological disturbances in disseminated sclerosis. Journal of Neurology, Neurosurgery and Psychiatry 29: 323–30.

Farmakides MN, Boone DR (1960) Speech problems of patients with multiple sclerosis. Journal of Speech and Hearing Disorders 25: 385–90.

Farmer A (1997) Spectrography. In Ball MJ, Code, C (eds) Instrumental Clinical Phonetics. London: Whurr Publishers Ltd.

Feinstein A, Kartsounis LD, Miller DH, Youl BD, Ron MA (1992) Clinically isolated lesions of the type seen in multiple sclerosis: a cognitive, psychiatric and MRI follow up study. Journal of Neurology, Neurosurgery and Psychiatry 55: 869–76.

Feinstein A, Ron M, Thompson A (1993) A serial study of psychometric and magnetic resonance imaging changes in multiple sclerosis. Brain 116: 569–602.

Felgenhauer K, Schadlich HJ, Nekic M, Ackermann R (1985) Cerebrospinal fluid antibodies: A diagnostic indicator for multiple sclerosis. Journal of the Neurological Sciences 71: 291–9.

Fex B, Kotby MN (1995) The accent method of voice therapy. In Kotby MN (ed.) Proceedings of the XXIII World Congress of the International Association of Logopedics and Phoniatrics: 103–6.

Filley CM, Heaton RK, Nelson LM, Burks RS, Franklin GM (1989) A comparison of dementia in Alzheimer's disease and multiple sclerosis. Archives of Neurology 46: 157–61.

Finlayson MA, Johnson KA, Reitan RM (1977) Relationship of level of education to neuropsychological measures in brain-damaged and non-brain-damaged adults. Journal of Consulting & Clinical Psychology 45: 402–11.

FitzGerald FJ, Murdoch BE, Chenery HJ (1987) Multiple sclerosis: associated speech and language disorders. Australian Journal of Human Communication Disorders 15: 15–33.

Fletcher SG (1970) Theory and instrumentation for quantitative measurement of nasality. Cleft Palate Journal 7: 601–9.

Flicker C, Feris S, Crook T, Bartus R (1987) Implications of memory and language dysfunction in the naming deficit of senile dementia. Brain and Language 31: 187–200.

Foley FW, Dince WM, Bedell JR, LaRocca NG, Kalb R, Caruso LS, Smith CR, Shnek ZM (1994) Psychoremediation of communication skills for cognitively impaired persons with multiple sclerosis. Journal of Neurologic Rehabilitation 8: 165–76.

Folkins JW, Abbs JH (1975) Lip and jaw motor control during speech: Response to resistive loading of the jaw. Journal of Speech and Hearing Research 18: 207–22.

Forrest K, Weismer G (1997) Acoustic analysis of dysarthric speech. In McNeil MR (ed.) Clinical Management of Sensorimotor Speech Disorders. New York, NY: Thieme Medical Publishers.

Francis DA (1993) The current therapy of multiple sclerosis. Journal of Clinical Pharmacy and Therapeutics 18: 77–84.

Franklin GM, Heaton RK, Nelson LM, Filley CM, Seibert C (1988) Correlation of neuropsychological and MRI findings in chronic progressive multiple sclerosis. Neurology 38: 1826–9.

Franklin GM, Nelson LM, Filley CM, Heaton RK (1989) Cognitive loss in multiple sclerosis: Case reports and review of the literature. Archives of Neurology 46: 162–7.

Frattali CM (1998a) Assessing functional outcomes: an overview. Seminars in Speech and Language 19: 209–19.

Frattali CM (1998b) Outcome measurement: definitions, dimensions and perspectives. In Frattali CM (ed.) Measuring Outcomes in Speech-Language Pathology. New York: Thieme.

Frattali CM, Thompson D, Holland A, Wohl C, Ferketic M (1995) American Speech-Language-Hearing Association Functional Assessment of Communication Skills for Adults. Rockville, MD: ASHA.

Frazier L, Rayner K (1987) Resolution of syntactic category ambiguities: eye movements in parsing lexically ambiguous sentences. Journal of Memory and Language 26: 505–26.

Freal JE, Kraft GH, Coryell JK (1984) Symptomatic fatigue in multiple sclerosis. Archives of Physical Medicine and Rehabilitation 65: 135–8.

Friedman JH, Brem H, Mayeux R (1983) Global aphasia in multiple sclerosis. Annals of Neurology 13: 222–3.

Froeschels E, Kastein S, Weiss D (1955) A method of therapy for paralytic conditions of the mechanisms of phonation, respiration, and glutination. Journal of Speech and Hearing Disorders 20: 365–70.

Frokjaer-Jensen B (1992) Data on air pressure, mean flow rate, glottal input and output energy, aerodynamic resistance, and glottal efficiency for normal healthy voices: a preliminary study. 22nd World Congress of International Association of Logopedics and Phoniatrics.

Gean-Marton AD, Gilbert-Vezina L, Marton KI, Stimac GK, Peyster RG, Taveras JM, Davis KR (1991) Abnormal corpus callosum: a sensitive and specific indicator of multiple sclerosis. Radiology 180: 215–21.

Gentner D (1983) Structure mapping: a theoretic framework for analogy. Cognitive Science 7: 155–70.

German DJ (1986) Test of Word Finding. National College of Education, Allen: DLM Teaching Resources.

Gibbon F, Dent H, Hardcastle W (1993) Diagnosis and therapy of abnormal alveolar stops in a speech-disturbed child using electropalatography. Clinical Linguistics and Phonetics 7: 247–67.

Gilbert HR, Potter CR, Hoodin R (1984) Laryngograph as a measure of vocal fold contact area. Journal of Speech and Hearing Research 27: 178–82.

Glosser G, Deser T (1990) Patterns of discourse production among neurological patients with fluent language disorders. Brain and Language 40: 67–88.

Glucksberg S (1989) Metaphors in conversation: how are they understood? why are they used? Metaphor and Symbolic Activity 4: 125–43.

Glucksberg S, Kreuz RJ, Rho S (1986) Context can constrain lexical access: implications for models of language comprehension. Journal of Experimental Psychology: Learning, Memory and Cognition 12: 323–35.

Goldstein G, Shelly CH (1975) Similarities and differences between psychological deficit in ageing and brain-damage. Journal of Gerontology 30: 448–55.

Goodglass H, Kaplan E (1979) Assessment of cognitive deficit in the brain injured patient. In Gazzaniga MS (ed.) Handbook of Behavioural Neurobiology: Vol 2 Neuropsychology. New York: Plenum Press: 3–22.

Goodglass H, Kaplan E (1983) Boston Diagnostic Aphasia Examination. In Goodglass H, Kaplan E (eds.) The Assessment of Aphasia and Related Disorders, 2nd edn. Philadelphia: Lea & Febiger.

Gordon WP (1985) Neuropsychologic assessment of aphasia. In Darby JK (ed.) Speech and Language Evaluation in Neurology: Adult Disorders. Orlando: Grune & Stratton: 161–96.

Gosselink R, Kovacs L, Decramer M (1999) Respiratory muscle involvement in multiple sclerosis. European Respiratory Journal 13: 449–54.

Griffiths C, Bough ID (1989) Neurologic diseases and their effect on voice. Journal of Voice 3(2): 148–56.

Grinker RR, Sahs AL (1966) Neurology, 6th edn. Springfield: Charles C. Thomas.

Gross Y, Schultz LE (1986) Intervention models in neuropsychology. In Uzell BP, Gross Y (eds.) Clinical Neuropsychology of Intervention. Boston: Martinus Nijhoff Publishing: 179–204.

Guilford AM, Nawojczyk DC (1988) Standardization of the Boston Naming Test at the kindergarten and elementary school levels. Language, Speech and Hearing Services in Schools 19: 395–400.

Haggard M P (1969) Speech waveform measurements in multiple sclerosis. Folia Phoniatrica 21: 307–12.

Hallpike JF, Adams WM, Tourtellotte WN (1983) Multiple Sclerosis. London: Chapman & Hall.

Hammen VL, Yorkston KM (1994) Effect of instruction on selected aerodynamic parameters in subjects with dysarthria and control subjects. In Till JA, Yorkston KM, Beukeleman DR (eds) Motor Speech Disorders: Advances in Assessment and Treatment. Baltimore: Paul H Brookes: 161–73.

Hanson DG, Gerratt BR, Karin RR, Berke GS (1988) Glottographic measures of vocal fold vibration: an examination of laryngeal paralysis. Laryngoscope 98: 541–8.

Hanson WR, Metter EJ (1980) DAF as instrumental treatment for dysarthria in progressive supranuclear palsy: a case report. Journal of Speech and Hearing Disorders 45: 268–75.

Hardcastle WJ, Morgan-Barry RA, Clark CJ (1985) Articulatory and voicing characteristics of adult dysarthric and verbal dyspraxic speakers: an instrumental study. British Journal of Disorders of Communication 20: 249–70.

Hardcastle WJ, Gibbon FE, Jones W (1991) Visual display of tongue-palate contact: electropalatography in the assessment and remediation of speech disorders. British Journal of Disorders of Communication 26: 41–74.

Hart RP, Kwentus JA, Leshner RT, Frazier R (1985) Information processing speed in Friedreich's ataxia. Annals of Neurology 17: 612–14.

Hartelius L, Svensson P (1994) Speech and swallowing symptoms associated with Parkinson's disease and multiple sclerosis: a survey. Folia Phoniatrica 46: 9–17.

Hartelius L, Svensson P, Bubach A (1993) Clinical assessment of dysarthria: performance on a dysarthria test by normal adult subjects, and by individuals with Parkinson's disease or with multiple sclerosis. Scandinavian Journal of Logopedics and Phoniatrics 18: 131–41.

Hartelius L, Nord L, Buder EH (1995) Acoustic analysis of dysarthria associated with multiple sclerosis. Clinical Linguistics and Phonetics 9: 95–120.

Hartelius L, Buder EH, Strand E (1997) Long-term phonatory instability in individuals with multiple sclerosis. Journal of Speech Language and Hearing Research 40: 1056–72.

Hartelius L, Wising C, Nord L (1997) Speech modification in dysarthria associated with multiple sclerosis: an intervention based on vocal efficiency, contrastive stress and verbal repair strategies. Journal of Medical Speech-Language Pathology 5(2): 113–40.

Hartelius L, Runmarker B, Anderson O (1999) Prevalence and characteristics of dysarthria in a multiple sclerosis incidence cohort in relation to neurological data. Folia Phoniatrica et Logopaedica.

Hartelius L, Runmarker B, Andersen O, Nord L (2000) Temporal speech characteristics of individuals with multiple sclerosis and ataxic dysarthria 'scanning speech' revisited. Folia Phoniatrica et Logopaedica (in press).

Hartley L (1990) Assessment of functional communication. In Tupper DE, Cicerone KD (eds) The Neuropsychology of Everyday Life, Volume 1: Assessment and Basic Competencies. Boston: Kluwer Academic Publishers: 125–67.

Hartley L (1995) Cognitive-Communication Abilities following Brain Injury: A Functional Approach. San Diego: Singular.

Hashimoto SA, Paty DW (1986) Multiple sclerosis. Disease-a-Month 32: 517–89.

Haughton VM, Zerrin-Yetkin F, Rao SM, Rimm AA, Fischer ME, Anne-Papke R, Breger RK, Khatri BO (1992) Quantitative MR in the diagnosis of multiple sclerosis. Magnetic Resonance in Medicine 26: 71–8.

Hauser SL, Fleischnick E, Weiner HL, Marcus D, Awdeh Z, Yunis EJ, Alper CA (1989) Extended major histocompatibility complex haplotypes in patients with multiple sclerosis. Neurology 39: 275–7.

Heaton RK, Nelson LM, Thompson DS, Burks JS, Franklin GM (1985) Neurological findings in relapsing remitting and chronic progressive multiple sclerosis. Journal of Consulting & Clinical Psychology 53: 103–10.

Helm NA (1979) Management of palilalia with a pacing board. Journal of Speech and Hearing Disorders 44: 350–3.

Herderschee D, Stam J, Derix MM (1987) Aphemia as a first symptom of multiple sclerosis. Journal of Neurology, Neurosurgery & Psychiatry 50: 499–500.

Hess CW, Mills KR, Murray NMF (1986) Measurement of central motor conduction in multiple sclerosis by magnetic brain stimulation. Lancet 2: 355–8.

Hess CW, Mills KR, Murray NMF, Schriefer TN (1987) Magnetic brain stimulation: central motor conduction studies in multiple sclerosis. Annals of Neurology 22: 744–52.

Hinchliffe FJ, Murdoch BE, Chenery HJ (1998) Towards a conceptualisation of language and cognitive impairment in closed-head injury: use of clinical measures. Brain Injury 12: 109–32.

Hinckley JJ, Craig HK (1992) A comparison of picture-stimulus and conversational elicitation contexts: responses to comments by adults with aphasia. Aphasiology 6: 257–72.

Hinton VA, Luschei ES (1992) Validation of a modern miniature transducer for measurement of interlabial contact pressure during speech. Journal of Speech and Hearing Research 35: 245–54.

Hirose H, Niimi S (1987) The relationship between glottal opening and the transglottal pressure differences during consonant production. In Baer T, Saski S, Harris K (eds) Laryngeal Function in Phonation and Respiration. Boston: College-Hill Press: 381–90.

Hirose H, Kiritani S, Ushijima T, Sawashima M (1978) Analysis of abnormal articulatory dynamics in two dysarthric patients. Journal of Speech and Hearing Disorders 43: 96–105.

Hixon TJ, Goldman M, Mead J (1973) Kinematics of the chest wall during speech production: volume displacements of the rib cage, abdomen and lung. Journal of Speech and Hearing Research 16: 78–115.

Hixon T, Hawley J, Wilson J (1982) An around the house device for the clinical determination of respiratory driving pressure: a note on making simple even simpler. Journal of Speech and Hearing Disorders 47: 413.

Hixon TJ, Putnam AH, Sharp JT (1983) Speech production with flaccid paralysis of the rib cage, diaphragm, and abdomen. Journal of Speech and Hearing Disorders 48: 315–27.

Hodge MM, Putnam-Rochet A (1989) Characteristics of speech breathing in young women. Journal of Speech and Hearing Research 32: 466–80.

Hodgson L (1993) Drug effects on speech. The Australian Communication Quarterly 12: 8.

Hogaboam TW, Perfetti CA (1975) Lexical ambiguity and sentence comprehension. Journal of Verbal Learning and Verbal Behaviour 14: 265–74.

Hoit JD, Hixon TJ (1986) Body type and speech breathing. Journal of Speech and Hearing Research 29: 313–24.

Hoit JD, Hixon TJ (1987) Age and speech breathing. Journal of Speech and Hearing Research 30: 351–66.

Hoit JD, Hixon TJ (1992) Age and laryngeal airway resistance during vowel production in women. Journal of Speech and Hearing Research 35: 309–13.

Honsinger MJ (1989) Midcourse intervention in multiple sclerosis: an inpatient model. AAC Augmentative and Alternative Communication 5: 71–3.

Horii Y (1983) An accelerometric measure as a physical correlate of perceived hypernasality in speech. Journal of Speech and Hearing Research 26: 476–80.

Howard RS, Wiles CM, Hirsch NP, Loh L, Spencer GT, Newsom DJ (1992) Respiratory involvement in multiple sclerosis. Brain 115: 479–94.

Huber SJ, Paulson GW, Shuttleworth EC, Chakeres D, Clapp LE, Pakalnis A, Weiss K, Rammohan K (1987) Magnetic resonance imaging correlates of dementia in multiple sclerosis. Archives of Neurology 44: 732–6.

Huber SJ, Bornstein RA, Rammohan KW, Christy JA, Chakeres DW, McGhee RB (1992) Magnetic resonance imaging correlates of neuropsychological impairment in multiple sclerosis. The Journal of Neuropsychiatry & Clinical Neurosciences 4: 152–8.

Hudson-Tennent LJ, Murdoch BE (1993) Retention of naming in children with an acquired language disorder subsequent to treatment for posterior fossa tumour. Journal of Medical Speech-Language Pathology 1: 95–105.

Huisingh R, Barrett M, Bagcen C, Orman O (1990). The Word Test – Revised. Ilinois: Lingui Systems.

Hutter C (1993) On the causes of multiple sclerosis. Medical Hypotheses 41: 93–6.

Hutters B, Brondsted K (1992) A simple nasal anemometer for clinical purposes. European Journal of Disorders of Communication 27: 101–19.

Hyman BT, Tranel D (1989) Hemianesthesia and aphasia: an anatomical and behavioural study. Archives of Neurology 46: 816–19.

Illes J (1989) Neurolinguistic features of spontaneous language production dissociate three forms of neurodegenerative disease: Alzheimer's, Huntington's and Parkinson's. Brain and Language 37: 628–42.

Isaac C, Li DK, Genton M, Jardine C, Grochowski E, Palmer M, Kastrukoff LF, Oger J, Paty DW (1988) Multiple sclerosis: a serial study using MRI in relapsing patients. Neurology 38: 1511–15.

Isshiki N, Honjow I, Morimoto M (1968) Effects of velopharyngeal incompetence upon speech. Cleft Palate Journal 5: 297.

Ivnik RJ (1978) Neuropsychological stability in multiple sclerosis. Journal of Consulting and Clinical Psychology 46: 913–23.

Izquierdo G, Campoy F, Mir J, Gonzalez M, Martinez-Parra C (1991) Memory and learning disturbances in multiple sclerosis: MRI lesions and neuropsychological correlation. European Journal of Radiology 13: 220–4.

Jacobs L, Johnson K P (1994) A brief history of the age of interferons as treatment of multiple sclerosis. Archives of Neurology 51: 1245–52.

Jacobs L, Goodkin DE, Rudick RA, Herndon R (1994) Advances in specific therapy for multiple sclerosis. Current Opinions in Neurology 7: 250–4.

Jambor KL (1969) Cognitive functioning in multiple sclerosis. British Journal of Psychiatry 115: 765–75.

Jennekens-Schinkel A, Laboyrie PM, Lanser JB, Van der Velde EA (1990) Cognition in patients with multiple sclerosis: after four years. Journal of Neurological Sciences 99: 229–47.

Jennekens-Schinkel A, Lanser JB, Van der Velde EA, Saunders EA (1990) Performances of multiple sclerosis patients in tasks requiring language and visuoconstruction: assessment of outpatients in quiescent disease stages. Journal of Neurological Sciences 95: 89–103.

Joanette Y, Goulet P (1990) Narrative discourse in right-brain-damaged right-handers. In Joanette Y, Brownell HH (eds.) Discourse Ability in Brain Damage. New York: Springer-Verlag: 131–53.

Johnson JA, Pring TR (1990) Speech therapy and Parkinson's disease: a review and further data. British Journal of Disorders of Communication 25: 183–94.

Jones J, Stone CA (1989) Metaphor comprehension by language learning disabled and normally achieving adolescent boys. Learning Disability Quarterly 12: 251–60.

Jordan FM, Ozanne AE, Murdoch BE (1990) Performance of closed head-injured children on a naming task. Brain Injury 4: 27–32.

Jorgensen C, Barrett M, Huisingh R, Sachman L (1981) The Word Test: a test of expressive vocabulary and semantics. Moline: LinguiSystems.

Jouandet M, Gazzaniga MS (1979) The Frontal Lobes. In Gazzaniga MS (ed.) Handbook of Behavioural Neurobiology: Vol. 2 Neuropsychology. New York: Plenum Press: 25–59.

Kaplan E, Goodglass H, Weintraub S (1983) The Boston Naming Test. Philadelphia: Lea and Febiger.

Kearns KP, Simmons NN (1988) Motor speech disorders: the dysarthrias and apraxia of speech. In Lass NJ, McReynolds IV, Northern JL, Yoder DE (eds.) Handbook of Speech-language Pathology and Audiology. Toronto: BC Decker: 592–621.

Keller E (1990) Speech motor timing. In Hardcastle WJ, Marchal A (eds.) Speech Production and Speech Modelling. Dordrecht: Kluwer Academic Publishers: 343–64.

Kennedy M, Murdoch BE (1990) Persistent word fluency deficits in patients with dominant hemisphere striato-capsular lesions: further evidence for a subcortical role in language. Australian Journal of Human Communication Disorders 18: 3–20.

Kent RD (1988) The dysarthric or apraxic client. In Yoder DE, Kent RD (eds.) Decision Making in Speech-language Pathology. Philadelphia: BC Decker: 156–7.

Kent RD, Netsell R (1975) A case study of an ataxic dysarthric: cineradiographic and spectrographic observations. Journal of Speech and Hearing Disorders 40: 115–34.

Kent RD, Read C (1992) The Acoustic Analysis of Speech. San Diego: Singular Publishing Co.

Kent RD, Rosenbek JC (1982) Prosodic disturbance and neurologic lesion. Brain and Language 15: 259–91.

Kent R, Netsell R, Bauer LL (1975) Cineradiographic assessment of articulatory mobility in the dysarthrias. Journal of Speech and Hearing Disorders 40: 467–80.

Kent RD, Netsell R, Abbs JH (1979) Acoustic characteristics of dysarthria associated with cerebellar disease. Journal of Speech and Hearing Research 22: 627–48.

Kent RD, Sufit RL, Rosenbek JC, Kent JF, Weismer G, Martin RE, Brooks BR (1991) Speech deterioration in amyotrophic lateral sclerosis: a case study. Journal of Speech and Hearing Research 34: 1269–75.

Kent RD, Kim H-H, Weismer G, Kent JF, Rosenbek JC, Brooks BR, Workinger M (1994) Laryngeal dysfunction in neurological disease: amyotrophic lateral sclerosis, Parkinson disease, and stroke. Journal of Medical Speech-Language Pathology 2(3): 157–75.

Kent RD, Kent JF, Rosenbek JC, Vorperian HK, Weismer G (1997) A speaking task analysis of the dysarthria in cerebellar disease. Folia Phoniatrica et Logopaedica 49: 63–82.

Kent-Braun JA, Sharma KR, Weiner MW, Miller RG (1994a) Effects of exercise on muscle activation and metabolism in multiple sclerosis. Muscle and Nerve 17: 1162–9.

Kent-Braun JA, Sharma KR, Weiner MW, Miller RG (1994b) Postexercise phosphocreatine resynthesis is slowed in multiple sclerosis. Muscle and Nerve 17: 835–41.

Kertesz A (1982) The Western Aphasia Battery. New York: Grune & Stratton.

Kirshner HS, Webb WG, Kelly MP (1984) The naming disorder of dementia. Neuropsychologia 22: 23–30.

Kirshner HS, Tsai SI, Runge VM, Price AC (1985) Magnetic resonance imaging and other techniques in the diagnosis of multiple sclerosis. Archives of Neurology 42: 859–63.

Klonoff H, Clark C, Oger J, Paty D, Li D (1991) Neuropsychological performance in patients with mild multiple sclerosis. Journal of Nervous and Mental Disease179: 127–31.

Knudson RJ, Lebowitz MD, Holberg CJ, Burrows B (1983) Changes in the normal maximal expiratory flow-volume curve with growth and aging. American Review of Respiratory Diseases 127: 725–34.

Kocsis JD, Waxman SG (1985) Demyelination: causes and mechanisms of clinical abnormality and functional recovery. In Vinken PJ, Bruyn GW, Klawans HL, Koetsier JC (eds.) Handbook of Clinical Neurology Volume 47. New York: Elsevier Science Publishing Company: 29–47.

Kohn SE, Goodglass H (1985) Picture naming in aphasia. Brain and Language 24: 266–83.

Kory RC, Callahan R, Boren HG (1961) The Veterans Administration-Army co-operative study of pulmonary function I: Clinical spirometry in normal men. American Journal of Medicine 30: 243–58.

Kotby MN (1995) The Accent Method of Voice Therapy. San Diego: Singular Publishing Group.

Kraft GH (1998) Rehabilitation principles for patients with multiple sclerosis. Journal of Spinal Cord Medicine 21: 117–20.

Kraft GH, Alquist AD, de Lateur BJ (1996) Effect of resistive exercise on physical function in multiple sclerosis (MS). Archives of Physical Medicine and Rehabilitation 33: 328–9.

Kuehn DP, Wachtel JM (1994) CPAP therapy for treating hypernasality following closed head injury. In Till JA, Yorkston KM, Beukelman, DR (eds) Motor Speech Disorders: Advances in Assessment and Treatment. Baltimore: Paul H Brookes: 207–12.

Kunzel H (1982) First applications of a biofeedback device for the therapy of velopharyngeal incompetence. Folia Phoniatrica 34: 92–100.

Kurtzke JF (1970) Clinical manifestations of multiple sclerosis. In Vinken PJ, Bruyn GW (eds) Handbook of Clinical Neurology: Vol. 9. Amsterdam: North Holland: 161–216.

Kurtzke JF (1983a) Epidemiology of multiple sclerosis. In Hallpike JF, Adams WM, Tourtellotte WW (eds) Multiple Sclerosis. Baltimore: Williams & Wilkins: 47–96.

Kurtzke JF (1983b) Rating neurologic impairment in multiple sclerosis: an expanded disability status scale (EDSS). Neurology 33: 1444–52.

LaBarge E, Edwards D, Knesevich JW (1986) Performance of normal elderly on the Boston Naming Test. Brain and Language 27: 380–4.

LaBarge E, Balota DA, Storandt M, Smith DS (1992) An analysis of confrontation naming errors in senile dementia of the Alzheimer type. Neuropsychology 6: 77–95.

Lane H, Perkell J, Svirsky M, Webster J (1991) Changes in speech breathing following cochlear implant in postlingually deafened adults. Journal of Speech and Hearing Research 34: 526–33.

Langmore SE, Lehman ME (1994) Physiologic deficits in the orofacial system underlying dysarthria in amyotrophic lateral sclerosis. Journal of Speech and Hearing Research 37: 28–37.

LeDorze G, Nespoulous J (1989) Anomia in moderate aphasia: problems in accessing the lexical representation. Brain and Language 37: 381–400.

Lehiste I (1977) Isochrony reconsidered. Journal of Phonetics 5: 253–63.

Lehman AJR, Tulley FM, Vrbova G, Dimitrijevic MR, Towle JA (1989) Muscle fatigue in some neurological disorders. Muscle and Nerve 12: 938–42.

Leibowitz S (1983) The immunology of multiple sclerosis. In Hallpike JF, Adams CWM, Tourtellotte WW (eds.) Multiple Sclerosis. Baltimore: Williams and Wilkins: 379–412.

Lethlean JB, Murdoch BE (1993) Language problems in multiple sclerosis. Journal of Medical Speech-Language Pathology 1: 47–59.

Lethlean JB, Murdoch BE (1994a) Naming errors in multiple sclerosis: Support for a combined semantic/perceptual deficit. Journal of Neurolinguistics 8: 207–23.

Lethlean JB, Murdoch BE (1994b) Naming in multiple sclerosis. Journal of Medical Speech Language Pathology 2: 43–56.

Lethlean JB, Murdoch BE (1997) Performance of subjects with multiple sclerosis on tests of high level language. Aphasiology 11: 39–57.

Levin HS (1990) Cognitive rehabilitation, unproven but promising. Archives of Neurology 47: 223–4.

Lieberman RR, Ellenberg M, Restum WH (1986) Aphasia associated with verified subcortical lesions: three case reports. Archives of Physiological and Medical Rehabilitation 67: 410–14.

Linebaugh CW (1983) Treatment of flaccid dysarthria. In Perkins W (ed.) Current Therapy of Communication Disorders: Dysarthria and Apraxia. New York: Thieme: 59–67.

Litvan I, Grafman J, Vendrell P, Martinez JM, Junque C, Vendrell JM and Barraquer-Bordas JL (1988) Multiple memory deficits in patients with multiple sclerosis: exploring the working memory system. Archives of Neurology 45: 607–10.

Luschei ES (1991) Development of objective standards of non-speech, oral strength and performance: an advocate's view. In Moore CA, Yorkston KM, Beukelman DR (eds.) Dysarthria and Apraxia of Speech: Perspectives on Management. Baltimore: Paul H Brookes : 3–14.

Lyon-Caen O, Jouvent R, Hauser S, Chaunu M, Benoit N, Widlocher D, Lhermitte F (1986) Cognitive function in recent onset demyelinating diseases. Archives of Neurology 43: 1138–41.

McAlpine D (1972) Multiple Sclerosis: A Reappraisal. Edinburgh: Churchill Livingstone.

McClosky DG (1977) General techniques and specific procedures for certain voice problems. In Cooper M, Cooper MH (eds.) Approaches to Vocal Rehabilitation. Springfield: Charles C Thomas: 138–52.

McDonald WI (1986) Pathophysiology of multiple sclerosis. In McDonald WI, Silberg DH (ed.) Multiple Sclerosis. London: Butterworth: 128–9.

McFarland DH, Smith A (1992) Effects of vocal task and respiratory phase on prephonatory chest wall movements. Journal of Speech and Hearing Research 35: 971–82.

McHenry MA, Minton JT, Wilson RL (1994) Increasing the efficiency of articulatory force testing of adults with traumatic brain injury. In Till JA, Yorkston KM, Beukelman DR (eds.) Motor Speech Disorders: Advances in Assessment and Treatment. Baltimore MD: Paul H Brookes: 135–46.

McLeod JG, Hammond SR, Hallpike JF (1994) Epidemiology of multiple sclerosis in Australia. Medical Journal of Australia 160: 117–22.

McNeil MR (ed.) (1997) Clinical Management of Sensorimotor Speech Disorders. New York NY: Thieme Medical Publishers.

McNeil MR, Prescott TE (1978) Revised Token Test. Baltimore: University Park Press.

McNeil MR, Weismer G, Adams S, Mulligan M (1990) Oral structure nonspeech motor control in normal dysarthric, aphasic and apraxic speakers: isometric force and static control. Journal of Speech and Hearing Research 33: 255–68

McWilliams BJ, Morris HC, Shelton RL (1990) Cleft Palate Speech. Philadelphia: BC Decker Inc.

Mahler ME (1992) Behavioural Manifestations Associated with Multiple Sclerosis. Psychiatric Clinics of North America 15: 427–38.

Manifold J, Murdoch B (1993) Speech breathing in young adults: effect of body type. Journal of Speech and Hearing Research 36: 657–71.

Margolin DI, Pate DS, Friedrich FJ, Elia E (1990) Dysnomia in dementia and in stroke patients: different underlying cognitive deficits. Journal of Clinical and Experimental Neuropsychology 12: 597–612.

Martin A, Fedio P (1983) Word production and comprehension in Alzheimer's disease: the breakdown of semantic knowledge. Brain and Language 19: 124–41.

Martin R, McFarland JF (1995) Immunological aspects of experimental allergic encephalomyelitis and multiple sclerosis. Critical Reviews in Clinical Laboratory Science 32: 121–82.

Matthews WB (1975) Paroxysmal symptoms in multiple sclerosis. Journal of Neurology, Neurosurgery and Psychiatry 38: 617–23.

Matthews, WB (1991) Clinical aspects. In Matthews WB, Compston A, Allen IV, Martyn CN (eds.) McAlpine's Multiple Sclerosis, 2nd edn. New York: Churchill Livingstone: 43–298.

Matthews WB, Compston A, Allen IV, Martyn CN (1991) McAlpine's Multiple Sclerosis. New York: Churchill Livingstone.

Mazaux JM, Richer E (1998) Rehabilitation after traumatic brain injury in adults. Disability and Rehabilitation 20: 435–47.

Mendez MF, Frey WH (1992) Multiple sclerosis dementia. Neurology 42: 696.

Mendozzi L, Pugnetti L, Saccani M, Motta A (1993) Frontal lobe dysfunction in multiple sclerosis as assessed by means of Lurian tasks: effects of age at onset. Journal of the Neurological Sciences 114 (Suppl.): 42–50.

Metter EJ (1987) Neuroanatomy and physiology of aphasia: evidence from positron emission tomography. Aphasiology 1: 3–33.

Metter EJ, Riege WR, Hanson WR, Jackson CA, Kempler D, Van Lancker D (1988) Subcortical structures in aphasia: analysis based on (F18)-fluoro-deoxyglucose positron emission tomography and computed tomography. Archives of Neurology 45: 1229–34.

Meulen V, Stephenson JR (1983) The possible role of viral infections in multiple sclerosis and other related demyelinating diseases. In Hallpike JF, Adams CWM, Tourtellotte WW (eds.) Multiple Sclerosis. Baltimore: Williams & Wilkins: 241–74.

Miller CJ, Daniloff R (1993) Airflow measurements: theory and utility of findings. Journal of Voice 7: 38–46.

Miller DH, Barkhof F, Berry I, Kappos L, Scotti G, Thompson AJ (1991) Magnetic resonance imaging in monitoring the treatment of multiple sclerosis: concerted action guidelines. Journal of Neurology, Neurosurgery and Psychiatry 54: 683–8.

Mills KR, Murray MF (1985) Corticospinal tract conduction time in multiple sclerosis. Annals of Neurology 18: 601–5.

Minden SL, Moes EJ, Orav J, Kaplan E, Reich P (1990) Memory impairment in multiple sclerosis. Journal of Clinical and Experimental Neuropsychology 12: 566–86.

Mitchell, G (1993) Update on multiple sclerosis therapy. Medical Clinics of North America 77: 231–49.

Mohr JP, Watters WC, Duncan GW (1975) Thalamic haemorrhage and aphasia. Brain and Language 2: 3–17.

Moll K L (1970) Objective measures of nasality. Cleft Palate Journal 7: 371–4.

Moncur JP, Brackett IP (1974) Modifying Vocal Behaviour. New York: Harper & Row.

Moon J, Lagu R (1987) Development of second-generation phototransducer for the assessment of velopharyngeal activity. Cleft Palate Journal 24: 240–3.

Murdoch BE, Chenery HJ, Bowler S, Ingram J (1989a) Respiratory function in Parkinson's subjects exhibiting a perceptible speech deficit: A kinematic and spirometric analysis. Journal of Speech and Hearing Disorders 54: 610–26.

Murdoch BE, Noble J, Chenery HJ, Ingram J (1989b) A spirometric and kinematic analysis of respiratory function in pseudobulbar palsy. Australian Journal of Human Communication Disorders 17: 21–35.

Murdoch BE, Theodoros DG, Stokes P, Chenery HJ (1993) Abnormal patterns of speech breathing in dysarthric speakers following severe closed head injury. Brain Injury 7: 295–308.

Murdoch BE, Thompson EC, Stokes PD (1994) Phonatory and laryngeal dysfunction following upper motor neurone vascular lesions. Journal of Medical Speech-Language Pathology 2: 177–89.

Murdoch BE, Attard M, Ozanne AE (1995) Impaired tongue strength and endurance in developmental verbal dyspraxia: a physiological analysis. European Journal of Communication Disorders 30: 51–64.

Murdoch BE, Sterling D, Theodoros DG (1995) Physiological rehabilitation of disordered speech breathing in dysarthric speakers following severe closed head injury. Paper presented at the Australian Society for the Study of Brain Impairment Conference, Hobart.

Murdoch BE, Spencer TJ, Theodoros DG, Thompson EC (1998) Lip and tongue function in multiple sclerosis: A physiological analysis. Motor Control 2: 148–60.

Nadeau SE (1991) Multi-infarct dementia, subcortical dementia and hydrocephalus. Southern Medical Journal 84 (Suppl. 1): 41–52.

Naeser MA, Alexander MP, Helm-Estabrooks N, Levine HL, Laughlin SA, Geschwind N (1982) Aphasia with predominantly subcortical lesion sites: Description of three capsular/putaminal aphasia syndromes. Archives of Neurology 39: 2–14.

Nemec RE, Cohen K (1984) EMG biofeedback in the modification of hypertonia in spastic dysarthria: a case report. Archives of Physical Medicine and Rehabilitation 65: 103–4.

Nesbit GM, Forbes GS, Scheithauer BW, Okazaki H, Rodriguez M (1991) Multiple sclerosis: Histopathologic and MR and/or CT in 37 cases of biopsy and three cases at autopsy. Radiology 180: 467–74.

Netsell R, Daniel B (1979) Dysarthria in adults: physiologic approach in rehabilitation. Archives of Physical Medicine and Rehabilitation 60: 502–8.

Netsell R, Hixon TJ (1978) A noninvasive method for clinically estimating subglottal air pressure. Journal of Speech and Hearing Disorders 63: 326–30.

Netsell R, Hixon TJ (1992) Inspiratory checking in therapy for individuals with speech breathing dysfunction. Journal of the American Speech and Hearing Association 34: 152.

Netsell R, Kent RD (1976) Paroxysmal ataxic dysarthria. Journal of Speech and Hearing Disorders 41: 93–109.

Netsell R, Rosenbek JC (1985) Treating the dysarthrias. In Darby J (ed.) Speech and Language Evaluation in Neurology: Adult disorders. Orlando: Grune & Stratton: 363–92.

Nicholas LE, Brookshire RH, MacLennan DL, Schumacher JG, Porrazzo SA (1989) Revised administration and scoring procedures for the BNT and norms for non-brain-damaged adults. Aphasiology 3: 569–80.

Noseworthy JH (1991) Therapeutics of multiple sclerosis. Clinical Neuropharmacology 14: 49–61.

Obler LK (1983) Language and brain dysfunction. In Segalowitz S J (ed.) Language Functions and Brain Organisation. New York: Academic Press: 267–82.

Obler LK, Dronkers NF, Koss E, Delis DC, Friedland RP (1986) Retrieval from semantic memory in Alzheimer's type dementia. Journal of Clinical and Experimental Neuropsychology 8: 75–92.

Olgiati R, Girr A, Hugi L, Haegi V (1989) Respiratory muscle training in multiple sclerosis: a pilot study. Schweiz Archives of Neurology and Psychiatry 140: 46–50.

Olmos-Lau BN, Ginsberg MD, Geller JB (1977) Aphasia in multiple sclerosis. Neurology 27: 623–6.

Onifer W, Swinney DA (1981) Accessing lexical ambiguities during sentence comprehension: Effects of frequency of meaning and contextual bias. Memory and Cognition 9: 225–36.

Osterman PO, Westerberg CE (1975) Paroxysmal attacks in multiple sclerosis. Brain 98: 189–202.

Parsons CL, Lambier J, Snow P, Couch D, Mooney L (1989) Conversational skills in closed head injury: Part 1. Australian Journal of Human Communication Disorders 17: 37–46.

Payne J C (1994) Communication Profile: A Functional Skills Survey. Arizona: Communication Skill Builders.

Perks WH, Lascelles RG (1976) Paroxysmal brain stem dysfunction as presenting feature of multiple sclerosis. British Medical Journal 2: 1175–6.

Peyser JM, Edwards KR, Poser CM, Filskov SB (1980) Cognitive function in patients with multiple sclerosis. Archives of Neurology 37: 577–9.

Peyser JM, Rao SM, LaRocca NG, Kaplan E (1990). Guidelines for neuropsychological research in multiple sclerosis. Archives of Neurology 47: 94–7.

Porter PB (1989) Intervention in end stage of multiple sclerosis: A case study. AAC Augmentative and Alternative Communication 5: 125–7.

Poser S (1978) Multiple sclerosis: an analysis of 812 cases by means of electronic data processing. New York: Springer-Verlag.

Poser CM (1994) The epidemiology of multiple sclerosis: A general overview. Annals of Neurology 36 (Suppl. 2): 180–93.

Poser CM, Paty DW, Scheinberg L, McDonald WI, Davis FA, Ebers GC, Johnson KP, Sibley WA, Silberberg DH, Tourtellotte WW (1983) New diagnostic criteria for multiple sclerosis. Annals of Neurology 13: 227–31.

Pozzilli C, Bastianello S, Padovani A, Passafiume D, Millefiorini E, Bozzao L, Fieschi C (1991) Anterior corpus callosum atrophy and verbal fluency in multiple sclerosis. Cortex 27: 441–5.

Pozzilli C, Passafiume D, Bernardi S, Pantano P, Incoccia C, Bastianello S, Bozzao L, Lenzi GL, Fieschi C (1991) SPECT, MRI and cognitive functions in multiple sclerosis. Journal of Neurology, Neurosurgery and Psychiatry 54: 110–15.

Pozzilli C, Gasperini C, Anzini A, Grasso M G, Ristori G, Fieschi C (1993) Anatomical and functional correlates of cognitive deficits in multiple sclerosis. Journal of the Neurological Sciences 115 (Suppl): 55–8.

Prater RJ, Swift RW (1984) Manual of Voice Therapy. Boston: Little, Brown & Co.

Prosek RA, Montgomery AA, Walden BE, Schwartz DM (1978) EMG biofeedback in the treatment of hyperfunctional voice disorders. Journal of Speech and Hearing Disorders 43: 282–94.

Prutting C, Kirchner D (1987) A clinical appraisal of the pragmatic aspects of language. Journal of Speech and Hearing Disorders 52: 105–19.

Pugnetti L, Mendozzi L, Motta A, Cattanco A, Biserni P, Caputo D, Cazzullo CL, Valsecchi F (1993) Magnetic resonance imaging and cognitive patterns in relapsing remitting multiple sclerosis. Journal of the Neurological Sciences 115 (Suppl): 59–65.

Rabins PV, Brooks BR, O'Donnell P, Pearlson GD, Moberg P, Julbelt B, Coyle P, Dalos N, Folstein MF (1986) Structural brain correlates of emotional disorders in multiple sclerosis. Brain 109: 585–97.

Raine CS (1977) The etiology and pathogenesis of multiple sclerosis: recent developments. Pathobiology Annual 7: 347–84.

Ramig LO (1992) The role of phonation in speech intelligibility: a review and preliminary data from patients with Parkinson's disease. In Kent RD (ed.) Intelligibility in Speech Disorders: Theory, measurement, and management. Philadelphia: John Benjamins Company: 119–55.

Ramig LO, Scherer RC (1989) Speech therapy for neurologic disorders of the larynx. In Blitzer A, Sasaki S, Fahn S et al. (eds.) Neurological Disorders of the Larynx. New York: Thieme Medical Publishers: 163–81.

Ramig LO, Mead C L, DeSanto l (1988) Voice therapy and Parkinson's disease. Journal of the American Speech and Hearing Association 30: 128.

Ramig LO, Titze IR, Scherer RC, Ringel SP (1988) Acoustic analysis of voices of patients with neurologic disease: rationale and preliminary data. Annals of Otology, Rhinology and Laryngology 97: 164–72.

Ramig LO, Scherer RC, Klasner ER, Titze IR, Horii Y (1990) Acoustic analysis of voice in amyotrophic lateral sclerosis; a longitudinal case study. Journal of Speech and Hearing Disorders 55: 2–14.

Ramig LO, Bonitati CM, Lemke JH, Horii Y (1994) Voice treatment for patients with Parkinson disease: development of an approach and preliminary efficacy data. Journal of Medical Speech-Language Pathology 2: 191–209.

Rao SM (1986) Neuropsychology of multiple sclerosis: a critical review. Journal of Clinical and Experimental Neuropsychology 8: 502–42.

Rao SM (1996) White matter disease and dementia. Brain and Cognition 31: 250–68.

Rao SM, Hammeke TA, McQuillen MP, Khatri BO, Lloyd D (1984) Memory disturbance in chronic progressive multiple sclerosis. Archives of Neurology 41: 625–31.

Rao SM, Glatt S, Hammeke TA, McQuillen MP, Khatri RO, Rhodes AM, Pollard S (1985) Chronic progressive multiple sclerosis: relationship between cerebral ventricular size and neuropsychological impairment. Archives of Neurology 42: 678–82.

Rao SM , Bernardin L, Leo GH, Ellington L, Ryan SB, Burg LS (1989) Cerebral disconnection in multiple sclerosis: relationship to atrophy of the corpus callosum. Archives of Neurology 46: 918–20.

Rao SM, Leo GJ, Haughton VM, St Aubin-Faubert P, Bernardin L (1989) Correlation of MRI with neuropsychological testing in multiple sclerosis. Neurology 39: 161–6.

Rao SM, St Aubin-Faubert P, Leo GJ (1989) Information processing speed in patients with multiple sclerosis. Journal of Clinical and Experimental Neuropsychology 11: 471–7.

Rao SM, Leo GJ, Bernardin L, Unverzagt F (1991) Cognitive dysfunction in multiple sclerosis: I. Frequency, patterns and predictions. Neurology 41: 658–91.

Rao SM, Grafman J, Di Giulio D, Mittenberg W, Bernardin L, Leo GJ, Luchetta T, Unverzagt F (1993) Memory dysfunction in multiple sclerosis: its relation to working memory, semantic encoding and implicit learning. Neuropsychology 7: 364–74.

Rice CL, Vollmer TL, Bigland-Ritchie B (1992) Neuromuscular responses of patients with multiple sclerosis. Muscle and Nerve 15: 1123–32.

Rivera VM (1986) Multiple sclerosis: Is the mystery beginning to unfold? Postgraduate Medicine 79: 217–32.

Robertson SJ, Thomson F (1984) Speech therapy in Parkinson's disease: a study of efficacy and long term effects of intensive treatment. British Journal of Disorders of Communication 19: 213–24.

Robin DA, Schienberg S (1990) Subcortical lesions and aphasia. Journal of Speech and Hearing Disorders 55: 90–100.

Robin DA, Somodi LB, Luschei ES (1991) Measurement of strength and endurance in normal and articulation disordered subjects. In Moore CA, Yorkston KM, Beukelman DR (eds) Dysarthria and Apraxia of Speech: Perspectives on management. Baltimore: Paul H Brookes: 173–84.

Robin DA, Goel A, Somodi, LB, Luschei ES (1992) Tongue strength and endurance: relation to highly skilled movements. Journal of Speech and Hearing Research 35: 1239–45.

Ron MA, Callanan MM, Warrington EK (1991) Cognitive abnormalities in multiple sclerosis: a psychometric and MRI study. Psychological Medicine 21: 59–68.

Ron MA, Feinstein A (1992) Multiple sclerosis and the mind. Journal of Neurology, Neurosurgery and Psychiatry 55: 1–3.

Rosenbek JC, LaPointe LL (1991) The dysarthrias: description, diagnosis, and treatment. In Johns D (ed.) Clinical Management of Neurogenic Communication Disorders. Boston: Little Brown & Co.: 97–152.

Rosenthal M (1995) Sheldon Berrol, MD Senior Lectureship: The ethics and efficacy of brain injury rehabilitation - myths, measurements and meaning. Journal of Head Trauma Rehabilitation 11: 88–95.

Rubow RT, Rosenbek JC, Collins M, Celesia GG (1984) Reduction in hemifacial spasm and dysarthria following EMG biofeedback. Journal of Speech and Hearing Disorders 49: 26–33.

Ruchkin DS, Grafman J, Krauss GL, Johnson R, Canoune H, Ritter W (1994) Event-related brain potential evidence for verbal working memory deficit in multiple sclerosis. Brain 117: 289–305.

Rudick RA (1992) The value of brain magnetic resonance imaging in multiple sclerosis. Archives of Neurology 49: 685–6.

Rudick R, Goodkin D (1992) Treatment of Multiple Sclerosis. Berlin: Springer.

Sadovnick AD (1994) Genetic epidemiology of multiple sclerosis: a survey. Annals of Neurology 36: S194–S203.

Sadovnick AD, Ebers GC, Wilson RW, Paty DW (1992) Life expectancy in patients with multiple sclerosis. Neurology 42: 991–4.

Sanderson K, Paulk J, Dodge G, Stephens S, Jones C, Dempsey R, Ross K, Muhlfeld A, Lall D, Freeman J, Croy J, Seikel JA, Madison C, Cooks NR, Brondos C (1996) Multiple sclerosis: presence of multiple consonant release bursts. Paper presented at the American Speech and Hearing Association Conference, Boston, MA.

Sandroni P, Walker C, Starr A (1992) Fatigue in patients with multiple sclerosis: Motor pathway conduction and event-related potentials. Archives of Neurology 49: 517–24.

Sandyk R (1994a) Improvement in word-fluency performance in patients with multiple sclerosis by electromagnetic fields. International Journal of Neuroscience 79: 75–90.

Sandyk R (1994b) Rapid normalization of visual evoked potentials by picotesla range magnetic fields in chronic progressive multiple sclerosis. International Journal of Neuroscience 77: 243–59.

Sandyk R (1995a) Chronic relapsing multiple sclerosis: A case of rapid recovery by application of weak electromagnetic fields. International Journal of Neuroscience 82: 223–42.

Sandyk R (1995b) Long term beneficial effects of weak electromagnetic fields in multiple sclerosis. International Journal of Neuroscience 83: 45–57.

Sandyk R (1995c) Resolution of dysarthria in multiple sclerosis by treatment with weak electromagnetic fields. International Journal of Neuroscience 83: 81–92.

Sandyk R (1996) Treatment with electromagnetic fields alters the clinical course of chronic progressive multiple sclerosis: a case report. International Journal of Neuroscience 88: 75–82.

Sandyk R (1997a) Immediate recovery of cognitive functions and resolution of fatigue by treatment with weak electromagnetic fields in a patient with multiple sclerosis. International Journal of Neuroscience 90: 59–74.

Sandyk R (1997b) Treatment with electromagnetic fields improves dual-task performance (talking while walking) in multiple sclerosis. International Journal of Neuroscience 92: 95–102.

Sarno M (1969) The Functional Communication Profile: Manual of Directions. New York: Institute of Rehabilitation Medicine.

Schiffer RB, Caine ED (1991) The interaction between depressive affective disorder and neuropsychological test performance in multiple sclerosis patients. Journal of Neuropsychiatry 3: 28–32.

Schwartz MF, Marin O, Saffran E (1979) Dissociations of language function in dementia: a case study. Brain & Language 7: 277–306.

Scolding NJ, Franklin RJM (1998) Axon loss in multiple sclerosis. Lancet 352: 340–1.

Scripture EW (1916) Records of speech in disseminated sclerosis. Brain 39: 445–77.

Scripture EW (1933) Diagnosis by soundtracks. Nature 132: 821–2.

Seikel JA, Richardson ML, Courtney-Dillman RA, Klaweno SL, Lawrence-Holmes K, Murphy SD, St.Hilaire-Murphy SM, Neal HL, Newton TG, Wilson ND, Madison CL, Cooke NR, Brondos CE (1996) Exacerbation in multiple sclerosis: Effect on formant frequencies. Paper presented at the American Speech and Hearing Association Conference, Seattle, WA.

Shaiman S (1989) Kinematic and electromyographic responses to perturbation of the jaw. Journal of the Acoustical Society of America 86: 78–88.

Sharma KR, Kent-Brown J, Mynhier MA, Weiner MW, Miller RG (1995) Evidence of an abnormal intramuscular component of fatigue in multiple sclerosis. Muscle and Nerve 18: 1403–11.

Sherwood L (1993) Human Physiology: From Cells to Systems, Second Edition. New York: West Publishing Co.

Shimamura AP, Salmon DP, Squire LR, Butters N (1987) Memory dysfunction and word priming in dementia and amnesia. Behavioural Neuroscience 101: 347–51.

Silverman FH (1993) Comprehensive bibliography on augmentative and alternative communication: a key to the AAC literature for clinicians and researchers. Greendale: CODI Publications.

Simmons NN (1983) Acoustic analysis of ataxic dysarthria: An approach to monitoring treatment. In Berry WR (ed.), Clinical dysarthria 283–94 San Diego: College-Hill Press: 283–94.

Simpson GB (1981) Meaning dominance and semantic context in the processing of lexical ambiguity. Journal of Verbal Learning & Verbal Behaviour 20: 120–36.

Simpson GB (1984) Lexical ambiguity and its role in models of word recognition. Psychological Bulletin 96: 316–40.

Simpson GB, Krueger MA (1991) Selective access of homograph meanings in sentence context. Journal of Memory & Language 30: 627–43.

Simpson MB, Till JA, Goff AM (1988) Long-term treatment of severe dysarthria: a case study. Journal of Speech and Hearing Disorders 53: 433–40.

Simpson GB, Peterson RR, Casteel MA, Burgess C (1989) Lexical and sentence context effects in word recognition. Journal of Experimental Psychology: Learning, memory and cognition 15: 88–97.

Smeltzer SC, Utell MJ, Rudick RA, Herndon RM (1988) Pulmonary function and dysfunction in multiple sclerosis. Archives of Neurology 45: 1245–9.

Smeltzer SC, Skurnick JH, Troiano R, Cook SD, Duran W, Lavietes MH (1992) Respiratory function in multiple sclerosis: Utility of clinical assessment of respiratory muscle function. Chest 101: 479–84.

Smeltzer SC, Lavietes MH, Cook S D (1996) Expiratory training in multiple sclerosis. Archives of Physical Medicine and Rehabilitation 77: 909–12.

Smith SR, Murdoch BE, Chenery HJ (1989) Semantic abilities in dementia of the Alzheimer type: I. Lexical semantics. Brain and Language 36: 314–24.

Smitheran JR, Hixon TJ (1981) A clinical method for estimating laryngeal airway resistance during vowel production. Journal of Speech and Hearing Disorders 46: 138–46.

Snodgrass JG (1984) Concepts and their surface representations. Journal of Verbal Learning & Verbal Behaviour 23: 3–22.

Solomon N, Hixon T J (1993) Speech breathing in Parkinson's disease. Journal of Speech and Hearing Research 36: 294–310.

Sperry EE, Klich RJ (1992) Speech breathing in senescent and younger women during oral reading. Journal of Speech and Hearing Research 35: 1246–55.

Spitzberg BH, Hurt HT (1987) The measurement of interpersonal skills in instructional contexts. Communication Education 36: 28–45.

Spreen O, Benton AL (1969) Neurosensory Centre Comprehensive Examination for Aphasia: Manual for Directions. Victoria BC: University of Victoria.

Stathopoulos ET, Sapienza C (1993) Respiratory and laryngeal function of women and men during vocal intensity variation. Journal of Speech and Hearing Research 36: 64–75.

Stevens KN, Kalikow DN, Willemain TR (1975) A miniature accelerometer for detecting glottal waveforms and nasalization. Journal of Speech and Hearing Research 18: 594–9.

Swirsky-Sacchetti T, Mitchell DR, Sewart J, Gonzales C, Lublin F, Knobler R, Field HL (1992). Neuropsychological and structural brain lesions in multiple sclerosis: a regional analysis. Neurology 42: 1291–5.

Tantucci C, Massucci M, Piperno R, Betti L, Grassi V, Sorbini CA (1994) Control of breathing and respiratory muscle strength in patients with multiple sclerosis. Chest 105: 1163–70.

Terrell BY, Ripich DN (1989) Discourse competence as a variable in intervention. Seminars in Speech and Language 10: 282–97.

Theodoros DG, Murdoch BE (1994) Laryngeal dysfunction in dysarthric speakers following severe closed head injury. Brain Injury 8: 667–84.

Theodoros DG, Murdoch BE, Stokes PD, Chenery HJ (1993) Hypernasality in dysarthric speakers following severe closed head injury: a perceptual and instrumental analysis. Brain Injury 7: 59–69.

Theodoros DG, Murdoch BE, Stokes PD (1995) A physiological analysis of articulatory dysfunction in dysarthric speakers following severe closed head injury. Brain Injury 9: 237–54.

Theodoros DG, Thompson EC (1998) Treatment of dysarthria. In Murdoch BE (ed.) Dysarthria: A Physiological Approach to Assessment and Treatment. Cheltenham: Stanley Thornes: 130–75.

Thompson EC, Murdoch BE (1995) Treatment of speech breathing disorders in dysarthria: a biofeedback approach. Paper presented at the Australian Association of Speech and Hearing Conference, Brisbane.

Thompson AF, Kennard C, Swash M, Summers B, Yuill GM, Shepherd DI, Roche S, Perkin GD, Loizou LA, Ferner R (1989) Relative efficacy of intravenous methylprednisolone and ACTH in the treatment of acute relapse in MS. Neurology 39: 969–71.

Thompson AJ, Kermode AG, Macmanus DG, Kendall BE, Kingsley DP, Moseley IF, McDonald WI (1990) Patterns of disease activity in multiple sclerosis: clinical and MRI study. British Medical Journal 300: 631–4.

Thompson AJ, Miller D, Youl B, Macmanus DG, Moore S, Kingsley D, Kendall B, Feinstein A, McDonald WI (1992) Serial gadolinium-enhanced MRI in relapsing remitting MS of varying disease duration. Neurology 42: 60–3.

Thompson EC, Murdoch BE, Stokes PD (1995a) Lip function in subjects with upper motor neuron type dysarthria following cerebrovascular accidents. European Journal of Disorders of Communication 30: 451–66.

Thompson EC, Murdoch BE, Stokes PD (1995b) Tongue function in subjects with upper motor neurone type dysarthria following cerebrovascular accidents. Journal of Medical Speech-Language Pathology 3: 27–40.

Thompson EC, Murdoch BE, Theodoros DG, Stokes PD (1996) Physiological assessment of interlabial contact pressures in normal and neurologically impaired adults. In Ponsford J, Snow P, Anderson V (eds.) Proceedings of the 5th Conference of the International Association for the study of Traumatic Brain Injury and the 20th Conference of the Australian Society for the Study of Brain Impairment. Brisbane: Academic Press: 259–66.

Thompson EC, Murdoch BE, Stokes PD (1997) Interlabial contact pressures during performance of speech tasks in young adults. Journal of Medical Speech-Language Pathology 5: 191–9.

Thompson-Ward EC, Murdoch BE, Stokes PD (1997) Biofeedback rehabilitation of speech breathing for an individual with dysarthria. Journal of Medical Speech-Language Pathology 5: 277–88.

Thompson-Ward EC, Theodoros DG (1998) Acoustic analysis of dysarthric speech. In Murdoch BE (ed.) Dysarthria: A Physiological Approach to Assessment and Treatment. Cheltenham UK: Stanley Thornes Publishers Ltd.

Thompson-Ward EC, Theodoros DG, Murdoch BE, Cahill L (1999) Use of a miniature lip transducer system in the assessment of patients with Parkinson's Disease. Journal of Medical Speech-Language Pathology 7:175–9.

Tienari PJ (1994) Multiple sclerosis: Multiple etiologies, multiple genes? Annals of Medicine 26: 259–69.

Till JA, Toye AR (1988) Acoustic phonetic effects of two types of verbal feedback in dysarthric speakers. Journal of Speech and Hearing Disorders 53: 449–58.

Titze IR, Durham PL (1987) Passive mechanisms influencing fundamental frequency control. In Baer T, Saski S, Harris K (eds.) Laryngeal Function in Phonation and Respiration. Boston: College-Hill Press: 304–19.

Tolosa ES, Alvarez R (1992) Differential diagnosis of cortical versus subcortical dementing disorders. Acta Neurologica Scandinavica 139: 47–53.

Troster AI, Salmon DD, McCullough D, Butters N (1989) A comparison of the category fluency deficits associated with Alzheimer's and Huntington's disease. Brain and Language 37: 500–13.

Twomey JA, Espir MLE (1980) Paroxysmal symptoms as the first manifestations of multiple sclerosis. Journal of Neurology, Neurosurgery and Psychiatry 43: 296–304.

Ulatowska HK, Chapman SB (1989) Discourse considerations for aphasia management. Seminars in Speech and Language 10: 298–314.

Vallar G, Papagno C, Cappa SF (1988) Latent dyphasia after left hemisphere lesions: a lexical-semantic and verbal memory deficit. Aphasiology 2: 463–78.

Van Demark D, Bzoch K, Daly D, Fletcher S, McWilliams B J, Pannbacker M, Weinberg B (1985) Methods of assessing speech in relation to velopharyngeal function. Cleft Palate Journal 22: 281–5.

Van den Burg W, Van Zomeren AH, Minderhoud JM, Prange AJ, Meijer SA (1987) Cognitive impairment in patients with multiple sclerosis and mild physical disability. Archives of Neurology 44: 494–501.

Van Gorp WG, Satz P, Evans-Kiersch M, Henry R (1986) Normative data on the BNT for a group of normal older adults. Journal of Clinical and Experimental Neuropsychology 8: 702–5.

Van Lancker D, Canter GF (1981) Idiomatic versus literal interpretations of ditropically ambiguous sentences. Journal of Speech and Hearing Research 24: 64–9.

van Oosten BW, Truyen L, Barkhof F, Polman CH (1995) Multiple sclerosis therapy. Drugs 49: 200–12.

Wallace GL, Holmes S (1993) Cognitive-linguistic assessment of individuals with multiple sclerosis. Archives of Physical Medicine and Rehabilitation 74: 637–43.

Wallesch CW (1985) Two syndromes of aphasia occurring with ischaemic lesions involving the left basal ganglia. Brain & Language 25: 357–61.

Wallesch CW, Papagno C (1988) Subcortical aphasia. In Rose FC, Whurr R, Wyke MA (eds.) Aphasia. London: Whurr Publishers: 256–87.

Weiner HL, Dau PC, Khatri BO, Petajan JH, Birnbaum G, McQuillan MP, Fasburg MT, Feldstein M, Orav EJ (1989) Double-blind study of true vs sham plasma exchange in patients treated with immunosuppression for acute attacks of multiple sclerosis. Neurology 39: 1143–49.

Weismer G (1984) Articulatory characteristics of parkinsonian dysarthria: segmental and phrase-level timing, spirantization, and glottal-supraglottal coordination. In McNeil MR, Rosenbek JC, Aronson AE (eds.) The Dysarthrias: Physiology, Acoustics, Perception, Management. San Diego: College-Hill Press: 101–30.

Whitaker JN, Mitchell GW (1997) Clinical features of multiple sclerosis. In Raine CS, McFarland HF, Tourtellotte WW (eds.) Multiple Sclerosis: Clinical and Pathogenic Basis. London: Chapman & Hall: 3–19.

White RF (1990) Emotional and cognitive correlates of multiple sclerosis. Journal of Neuropsychiatry & Clinical Neurosciences 2: 422–8.

Wiig EH, Secord W (1985) Test of Language Competence. Columbus: Merril.

Wiig EH, Secord E (1989) Test of Language Competence – Expanded. Ohio: Charles E. Merrill.

Wiig EH, Semel EM (1974) Development of comprehension of logico-grammatical sentences by grade school children. Perceptual and Motor Skills 38: 175–6.

Wikstrom M, Kinnunen E, Porras J (1984) The age-specific prevalence ratio of familial multiple sclerosis. Neuroepidemiology 3: 74–82.

Winholz WS, Ramig LO (1992) Vocal tremor analysis with the vocal demodulator. Journal of Speech and Hearing Research 35: 562–73.

Winkworth AL, Davis PJ, Adams RD, Ellis E (1995) Breathing patterns during spontaneous speech. Journal of Speech and Hearing Research 38: 124–44.

Winner E (1988) The point of words: Children's understanding of metaphor and irony. Cambridge: Havard University Press.

World Health Organization (1980) The international classification of diseases 10th revision (ICD-10). Chapter V: Mental, behavioural and developmental disorders. Geneva: WHO typescript document MNH/MEP/87.1: 25–31.

Worrall L, Burtenshaw EJ (1990) Frequency of use and utility of aphasia tests. Australian Journal of Human Communication Disorders 18: 53–63.

Yorkston KM, Beukelman DR (1978) A comparison of techniques for measuring intelligibility of dysarthric speech. Journal of Communication Disorders 11: 499–512.

Yorkston KM, Beukelman DR (1981) Assessment of Intelligibility of Dysarthric Speech. Austin: Pro-Ed.

Yorkston KM, Beukelman DR, Bell KR (1988) Clinical Management of Dysarthric Speakers. Boston: College-Hill Press.

Yorkston KM, Miller RM, Strand EA (1995) Multiple sclerosis. In Yorkston KM, Miller RM, Strand EA (eds.) Management of Speech and Swallowing in Degenerative Diseases. Tucson: Communication Skill Builders: 179–206.

Zemlin WR (1962) A comparison of the periodic function of vocal fold vibration in a multiple sclerotic and a normal population. Unpublished doctoral thesis, University of Minnesota.

Zemlin WR (1988) Speech and Hearing Science: Anatomy and Physiology. Englewood Cliffs, New Jersey: Prentice-Hall Inc.

Ziegler W, Hartmann E, Hoole P (1993) Syllabic timing in dysarthria. Journal of Speech and Hearing Research 36: 683–93.

Zwirner P, Murry T, Woodson GE (1991) Phonatory function of neurologically impaired patients. Journal of Communication Disorders 24: 287–300.

Index

abdominal binding/girdling 85
abdominal paradoxing 76
abdominal support during exhalation 84
absurdities 202
accelerometry 93
accent method, in breathing exercises 84, 88
accessing deficit, lexical 145–6
acoustic analysis 30–1, 37, 46
    case study 41–5
    contrastive stress sentences 43–4
    passage reading 43
    verbal repairs 44–5
    in neurological disorders 31–3
    phonatory characteristics 30
    spectral characteristics 30
    temporal characteristics 30
adrenocorticotrophic hormone (ACTH) 8
Aerophone II voice function analyser 69
age, and language abilities 159
agraphia 112
air flow transducers 88, 95
alexia 112
alphabet boards 97
Alzheimer's disease 144, 146, 147
amantadine 9
ambiguity 135–8, 189, 202
    processing models 136–7
    types of 136
American Speech-Language-Hearing Association (ASHA) Functional Assessment of Communication Skills for Adults 205
amyotrophic lateral sclerosis (ALS) 28, 31, 58

Analysis of Monologic Discourse 205
Analysis of Topic 205
anemometer, warm/hot-wire 61, 69
anomia 124–5, 125
anticholinergic medication 9
antidepressants 9
    tricyclic 141–2, 160
antiepileptics 142, 160
antispastic agents 8
antonyms 135, 188
aphasia, case studies 111–12
Aphasia Screening Test (AST) 113
aphasia test batteries 113–15
Arizona Battery for Communication Disorders 115
articulation
    imprecise 20, 21, 22, 23, 29, 37–8, 59
    sudden breakdown 23
articulatory dysfunction 47–8, 48–59
    perceptual features 48
    physiological assessment 48–51
    physiological features 51–9
    treatment 90–1, 94–5
    behavioural techniques 94
    instrumental techniques 95
ASHA (American Speech-Language-Hearing Association) Functional Assessment of Communication Skills for Adults 205
Assessment of Intelligibility of Dysarthric Speech (ASSIDS) 19
AST (Aphasia Screening Test) 113
ataxia 8–9
    laryngeal 39
ataxic dysarthria 33, 35, 36

253